T0249426

Rehabilitation Therapy

Editor

MOLLY J. FLAHERTY

VETERINARY CLINICS OF NORTH AMERICA: SMALL ANIMAL PRACTICE

www.vetsmall.theclinics.com

July 2023 • Volume 53 • Number 4

ELSEVIER

1600 John F. Kennedy Boulevard • Suite 1800 • Philadelphia, Pennsylvania, 19103-2899
http://www.vetsmall.theclinics.com

**VETERINARY CLINICS OF NORTH AMERICA: SMALL ANIMAL PRACTICE Volume 53, Number 4
July 2023 ISSN 0195-5616, ISBN-13: 978-0-443-18228-0**

Editor: Stacy Eastman
Developmental Editor: Axell Ivan Jade Purificacion

Veterinary Clinics of North America: Small Animal Practice (ISSN 0195-5616) is published bimonthly by Elsevier Inc., 360 Park Avenue South, New York, NY 10010-1710. Months of issue are January, March, May, July, September, and November. Business and Editorial Offices: 1600 John F. Kennedy Blvd., Ste. 1800, Philadelphia, PA 19103-2899. Customer Service Office: 3251 Riverport Lane, Maryland Heights, MO 63043. Periodicals postage paid at New York, NY and additional mailing offices. Subscription prices are $387.00 per year (domestic individuals), $844.00 per year (domestic institutions), $100.00 per year (domestic students/residents), $488.00 per year (Canadian individuals), $1049.00 per year (Canadian institutions), $528.00 per year (international individuals), $1049.00 per year (international institutions), $100.00 per year (Canadian students/residents), and $220.00 per year (international students/residents). To receive student/resident rate, orders must be accompanied by name of affiliated institution, date of term, and the *signature* of program/residency coordinator on institution letterhead. Orders will be billed at individual rate until proof of status is received. Foreign air speed delivery is included in all *Clinics* subscription prices. All prices are subject to change without notice. **POSTMASTER:** Send address changes to *Veterinary Clinics of North America: Small Animal Practice*, Elsevier Health Sciences Division, Subscription Customer Service, 3251 Riverport Lane, Maryland Heights, MO 63043. Customer Service (orders, claims, online, change of address): Elsevier Periodicals Customer Service, Elsevier Health Sciences Division Subscription **Customer Service 3251 Riverport Lane Maryland Heights, MO 63043. Tel: 1-800-654-2452 (U.S. and Canada); 314-447-8871 (outside U.S. and Canada). Fax: 314-447-8029. E-mail: journalscustomerservice-usa@elsevier.com (for print support); journalsonlinesupport-usa@elsevier.com (for online support).**

Reprints. For copies of 100 or more of articles in this publication, please contact the Commercial Reprints Department, Elsevier Inc., 360 Park Avenue South, New York, NY 10010-1710. Tel.: 212-633-3874; Fax: 212-633-3820; E-mail: reprints@elsevier.com.

Veterinary Clinics of North America: Small Animal Practice is also published in Japanese by Inter Zoo Publishing Co., Ltd., Aoyama Crystal-Bldg 5F, 3-5-12 Kitaaoyama, Minato-ku, Tokyo 107-0061, Japan.

Veterinary Clinics of North America: Small Animal Practice is covered in *Current Contents/Agriculture, Biology and Environmental Sciences, Science Citation Index, ASCA, MEDLINE/PubMed (Index Medicus), Excerpta Medica, and BIOSIS.*

Contributors

EDITOR

MOLLY J. FLAHERTY, DVM, CCRP, CVA, CVSMT, CVPP
Director of Rehabilitation Medicine, Department of Clinical Sciences and Advanced Medicine, Ryan Veterinary Hospital, School of Veterinary Medicine, University of Pennsylvania, Philadelphia, Pennsylvania, USA

AUTHORS

RIA ACCIANI, MPT, CCRP
Advanced Canine Rehabilitation Center, Warren, New Jersey, USA

JERET BENSON, DVM, MS
Red Sage Integrative Veterinary Partners, Fort Collins, Colorado, USA

JESSICA BUNCH, DVM, CCRT, CVA
Associate Professor, Integrative Veterinary Medicine and Rehabilitation, College of Veterinary Medicine, Washington State University, Pullman, Washington, USA

BRITTANY JEAN CARR, DVM, CCRT
Diplomate, American College of Veterinary Sports Medicine and Rehabilitation; The Veterinary Sports Medicine and Rehabilitation Center

KELLY DEABOLD, DVM, CCRV, CVA
Resident, Department of Comparative, Diagnostic and Population Medicine, College of Veterinary Medicine, University of Florida, Gainesville, Florida, USA

LAURIE EDGE-HUGHES, BScPT, MAnimST, CCRT, CAFCI
The Canine Fitness Centre Ltd, Calgary, Alberta, Canada

BRIAN D. FARR, DVM, MSTR
Diplomate, American College of Veterinary Preventive Medicine; Department of Defense Military Working Dog Veterinary Service, Joint Base San Antonio–Lackland Air Force Base, San Antonio, Texas, USA

MOLLY J. FLAHERTY, DVM, CCRP, CVA, CVSMT, CVPP
Director of Rehabilitation Medicine, Department of Clinical Sciences and Advanced Medicine, Ryan Veterinary Hospital, School of Veterinary Medicine, University of Pennsylvania, Philadelphia, Pennsylvania, USA

LINDSEY FRY, DVM
Diplomate, American College of Veterinary Sports Medicine and Rehabilitation; Fort Collins, Colorado, USA

AMBER IHRKE, DVM, CCRT, CVA, CVSMT, CVPP
Diplomate, American College of Veterinary Sports Medicine and Rehabilitation; Veterinary Sports Medicine and Rehabilitation of Homer Glen, Homer Glen, Illinois, USA

AMY LEE KRAMER, DPT, CCRT
Beach Animal Rehabilitation Center, Torrance, California, USA

ROSEMARY J. LOGIUDICE, DVM, CCRT, CVA, CVSMT, FCoAC
Diplomate, American College of Veterinary Sports Medicine and Rehabilitation; Owner, Animal Rehabilitation Therapy and Sports Medicine, Yorkville, Illinois, USA; Senior Faculty, Healing Oasis Wellness Center, Sturtevant, Wisconsin, USA

CAROLINA MEDINA, DVM
Diplomate, American College of Veterinary Sports Medicine and Rehabilitation; Certified Veterinary Acupuncturist (CVA), Certified Veterinary Pain Practitioner (CVPP), Elanco Animal Health, Greenfield, Indiana, USA

ERIN MISCIOSCIA, DVM, CVA
Diplomate, American College of Veterinary Sports Medicine and Rehabilitation; Clinical Assistant Professor, Department of Comparative, Diagnostic and Population Medicine, College of Veterinary Medicine, University of Florida, Gainesville, Florida, USA

CHRISTINA MONTALBANO, VMD, CCRP, CVA
Diplomate, American College of Veterinary Sports Medicine and Rehabilitation; Clinical Assistant Professor, NorthStar VETS, Robbinsville, New Jersey, USA

CYNTHIA M. OTTO, DVM, PhD
Diplomate, American College of Veterinary Emergency and Critical Care; Diplomate, American College of Veterinary Sports Medicine and Rehabilitation; Penn Vet Working Dog Center, Clinical Sciences and Advanced Medicine, School of Veterinary Medicine, University of Pennsylvania, Philadelphia, Pennsylvania, USA

THERESA E. PANCOTTO, DVM, MS, CCRP
Diplomate, American College of Veterinary Internal Medicine(Neurology); Neurologist/ Neurosurgeon, Specialists in Companion Animal Neurology, USA

ARIELLE PECHETTE MARKLEY, DVM, cVMA, CVPP, CCRT
Diplomate, Academy of Integrative Pain Management; Assistant Professor, Department of Clinical Sciences, Sports Medicine and Rehabilitation, The Ohio State University College of Veterinary Medicine, Columbus, Ohio, USA

MEGHAN T. RAMOS, VMD
Penn Vet Working Dog Center, Clinical Sciences and Advanced Medicine, School of Veterinary Medicine, University of Pennsylvania, Philadelphia, Pennsylvania, USA

PEDRO LUIS RIVERA, DVM, FACFN
FCoAC, Diplomate, American College of Veterinary Sports Medicine and Rehabilitation; Co-owner and Program Director, Healing Oasis Wellness Center, Co-owner, Healing Oasis Veterinary Hospital, Sturtevant, Wisconsin, USA

JESSICA RYCHEL, DVM
Diplomate, American College of Veterinary Sports Medicine and Rehabilitation; Fort Collins, Colorado, USA

Contents

> Pain recognition, assessment, and management is a primary focus and an integral part of veterinary rehabilitation. Evidence-based pain mitigation protocols will use both pharmacologic tools and nonpharmacologic methods to create a customized, safe, and effective treatment plan. A multimodal, patient-centered approach will allow for the best outcomes for pain relief and improved quality of life.

> Manual therapy is a cornerstone of physical therapy and canine physical rehabilitation. Although veterinary literature has tackled the topic of manual therapy treatments in animal patients, less attention has been paid to the assessment techniques and clinical reasoning skills that guide a practitioner toward determining if, when, and where manual therapies will be most effective. This article tackles the topics of clinical reasoning, the functional diagnosis, observational skills, and physical evaluation techniques that serve as prerequisites to the use of manual therapeutics.

 Video content accompanies this article at http://www.vetsmall. theclinics.com.

> Veterinary rehabilitation is a multimodal diagnostic and treatment approach that is recommended and provided to patients daily. One therapeutic modality that may be beneficial (diagnostically and therapeutically) is veterinary spinal manipulative therapy or animal chiropractic (AC). AC is a receptor-based health-care modality being provided more frequently in veterinary practices. All clinicians should strive to understand the mode of action, indications, contraindications, how it affects the patient from the neuro-anatomical and biomechanical point of view, and most importantly, when not to provide the requested modality, as further diagnostics may be indicated.

Extracorporeal shockwave therapy (ESWT) is a noninvasive treatment that involves the transcutaneous delivery of high-energy sound waves into tissue creating therapeutic effects. Shockwaves are nonlinear, high-pressure, high-velocity acoustic waves characterized by low tensile amplitude, short rise time to peak pressure, and a short duration (less than 10 milliseconds). ESWT has been shown to increase the expression of cytokines and growth factors leading to decreased inflammation, neovascularization, and cellular proliferation; activation of osteogenesis by osteoblast differentiation and then by increased proliferation; inhibition of cartilage degeneration and rebuilding of subchondral bone; and increased serotonin in the dorsal horn and descending inhibition of pain signals. Musculoskeletal conditions that can benefit from ESWT include osteoarthritis, tendinopathies, fracture/bone healing, and wound healing.

Photobiomodulation therapy, also commonly known as laser therapy, continues to grow in popularity in veterinary medicine. It is the use of red and near-infrared light to simulate healing, relieve pain, and reduce inflammation. The potential variety of conditions for which it can be used as an adjunctive, non-invasive modality has propelled its use in both veterinary rehabilitation, sports medicine, and general practice. In the last decade, clinical research has grown with increasing evidence for efficacy for some conditions but mixed to limited in others and many conditions not represented.

Regenerative medicine is used in the canine to optimize tissue healing and treat osteoarthritis and soft tissue injuries. Rehabilitation therapy is also often implemented in the treatment and management of musculoskeletal conditions in the canine. Initial experimental studies have shown that regenerative medicine and rehabilitation therapy may work safely and synergistically to enhance tissue healing. Although additional study is required to define optional rehabilitation therapy protocols after regenerative medicine therapy in the canine, certain fundamental principles of rehabilitation therapy still apply to patients treated with regenerative medicine.

Agility is a physically demanding sport, and injuries are common. An understanding of the common clinical presentations, frequent injuries, and risk factors for injury is critical when seeing this population of patients in practice. Shoulder injuries and other soft tissue injuries including iliopsoas muscle strains are commonly seen. The Border Collie seems to be at higher risk of developing agility-related injuries. The key to rehabilitation of the agility dog is accurate and expedient diagnosis of the injury, which often involves advanced diagnostics such as musculoskeletal ultrasound, arthroscopy, and/or MRI.

Degenerative myelopathy is an inherited, progressive, neurodegenerative disorder affecting the spinal cord of dogs. There is no treatment of the disease. Physical rehabilitation is the only intervention that slows progression and prolongs quality of life. Further studies are needed to develop advanced treatment options and to better characterize the use of complementary therapeutic modalities in palliative care for these patients.

 Video content accompanies this article at http://www.vetsmall. theclinics.com.

Therapy exercises can help to optimize the outcome for dogs following cranial cruciate ligament repair surgery. This article focuses on land exercises that can be done with minimal equipment in home or in clinic. The first 8 weeks of recovery are covered including therapy and basic exercises for each phase.

This article highlights the differences between working dog careers, unique protocols associated with health care of a working dog and provides a practical guide to creating and managing a return-to-work program. The rehabilitative approach to a working dog consists of four distinct sequential phases: activity restriction, rehabilitation, return-to-work, and maintenance. The timeline through each phase is dependent on the degree of injury, treatment intervention, prior health status of the dog, and compliance of the handler. Return-to-work for a working dog is considered a success if the dog can perform all career-related activities safely and proficiently.

Feline osteoarthritis is common; despite vague clinical signs, it can result in mobility impairment and quality of life concerns. An integrative approach to management may include analgesic medications, dietary modifications, nutraceuticals, environmental modifications, physical rehabilitation, acupuncture, and regenerative medicine. Management of concurrent disease and consideration for patient tolerance and owner compliance are critical in formulating a treatment plan in cats with osteoarthritis.

Palliative care is a unique area of veterinary medicine, where primary goals include maintaining quality of life, as opposed to treating with a curative intent. Using the disablement model and client partnership allows for the development of a function-targeted treatment plan individualized to patient and family needs. Rehabilitation modalities, especially when combined with adaptive pain management, are well-suited to palliative care because they can greatly enhance a patient's ability to achieve improved function and quality of life. These areas join in a concept called palliative rehabilitation which combines the unique needs of these patients and the tools accessible to the rehabilitation practitioner.

VETERINARY CLINICS OF NORTH AMERICA: SMALL ANIMAL PRACTICE

SERIES OF RELATED INTEREST

Veterinary Clinics: Exotic Animal Practice
https://www.vetexotic.theclinics.com/
Advances in Small Animal Care
https://www.advancesinsmallanimalcare.com/

THE CLINICS ARE NOW AVAILABLE ONLINE!
Access your subscription at:
www.theclinics.com

Preface

Veterinary Rehabilitation Updates: From Pain Management to Healing and Function

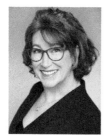

Molly J. Flaherty, DVM, CCRP, CVA, CVSMT, CVPP
Editor

It is a great honor to act as guest editor and author for the *Veterinary Clinics of North America: Small Animal Practice* issue on Rehabilitation Therapy. Being a part of the field of veterinary rehabilitation has been a joy in my career. It provides so many benefits to our patients, including pain relief, mobility, quality of life, improved health, and enhancement of the human animal bond. The last rehabilitation therapy–dedicated issue was in 2015, and the field continues to grow by leaps and bounds, attracting practitioners all over the world passionate about their work.

There are many facets of veterinary medicine that overlap with rehabilitation, and this issue has something for everyone. The topics recruited include those of current interest and questions most often asked. Articles in this issue hold a wide range of appeal for readers, including pain management, canine- and feline-focused topics, sporting and working dogs, modalities, manual and exercise therapy, alternative medicine, and palliative care. I think you will find a breadth of information for those just learning more about rehab, those incorporating rehab into practice, and the experienced rehabilitation practitioner alike. More research in rehabilitation continues to emerge, and evidence-based reviews are incorporated throughout the articles.

This issue begins with a review of pain management, reflecting this as foremost in rehabilitation therapy and a significant role in what we provide as rehabilitation practitioners. The following articles reinforce this through discussion of various modalities, treatments, therapies, medication, and supplements. All aspects of rehabilitation unite to address pain in a multimodal approach.

I wish to thank all the authors who contributed to this issue for their outstanding expertise. With their collective knowledge, we can present the opportunity to learn and grow in our practice. It is my hope that this will have a positive impact in the field

Vet Clin Small Anim 53 (2023) xi–xii
https://doi.org/10.1016/j.cvsm.2023.04.001
0195-5616/23/© 2023 Published by Elsevier Inc.

vetsmall.theclinics.com

of veterinary rehabilitation therapy and promote insight of what rehabilitation therapy can provide for our patients.

Molly J. Flaherty, DVM, CCRP, CVA, CVSMT, CVPP
Department of Clinical Sciences and
Advanced Medicine
School of Veterinary Medicine
University of Pennsylvania

Department of Clinical Sciences
Ryan Veterinary Hospital
3900 Delancey Street
Philadelphia, PA 19104, USA

E-mail address:
mollyfl@vet.upenn.edu

Multimodal Approach to Pain Management in Veterinary Rehabilitation

Amber Ihrke, DVM, DACVSMR

KEYWORDS

- Multimodal pain management • Veterinary rehabilitation • Pharmacology
- Pain physiology • Therapeutic exercise

KEY POINTS

- Pain recognition, assessment, and treatment is essential for successful patient outcome.
- Strive for a multimodal approach to pain management, as transmission of pain is complex, thereby interrupting pain via multiple pathways has been shown to be more effective than relying on a single mechanism.
- Evidence-based pain management protocols will use both pharmacologic and nonpharmacologic tools.
- Manual therapy, therapeutic exercises, and physical modalities are the cornerstone of a veterinary rehabilitation pain management plan.

INTRODUCTION

Veterinary rehabilitation is a science dedicated to improving maximal movement and functional mobility for our patients. Pain recognition, assessment, and treatment is essential for successful patient outcome, and a pain management strategy should be part of every treatment protocol. The goal of this article is to review the multimodal approach of common pharmacologic and nonpharmacologic interventions for pain management used in a rehabilitation therapy setting.

PHYSIOLOGY OF PAIN

Pain can be defined as "an aversive sensory and emotional experience representing an awareness by the animal of damage or threat to the integrity of its tissues; it changes the animal's physiology and behavior to reduce or avoid damage, to reduce the likelihood of recurrence and to promote recovery."[1] In common terms, pain can be described as acute or chronic. Acute pain occurs in response to tissue damage that

Diplomate of American College of Sports Medicine and Rehabilitation, Veterinary Sports Medicine & Rehabilitation of Homer Glen, 13726 W. 159th Street, Homer Glen, IL, 60491, USA
E-mail address: aihrke@vsmrhg.com

Vet Clin Small Anim 53 (2023) 731–742
https://doi.org/10.1016/j.cvsm.2023.02.006
0195-5616/23/© 2023 Elsevier Inc. All rights reserved.

vetsmall.theclinics.com

resolves over a relatively short period of time (days or weeks), disappears with healing, and tends be self-limiting.[2,3] Chronic pain persists beyond the expected healing time when nonmalignant in origin (weeks or months).[3] Nociception is the process where the nervous system detects potentially harmful stimulus and transmit the information to the brain, which when combined with an emotional component results in pain.[4] The process where nociception is recognized as pain involves the following:

1. Transduction: translation of mechanical, chemical, or thermal noxious stimuli into a nociceptive impulse.[3,5]
2. Transmission: propagation of action potential by primary afferent neurons to carry sensory information to the dorsal horn of the spinal cord.[5]
3. Modulation: nociceptive information is amplified or dampened in the spinal cord with input from ascending and descending pathways.[5]
4. Projection: nociceptive information is conveyed from the spinal cord to the somato-sensory cortex of the brain.[3,5]
5. Perception: integration of sensory information by the cortex to have a conscious, emotional experience of pain and produce a response.[3,5] The cerebral cortex exerts a top-down control and modulates pain.[6]

Pathophysiology of Pain

Adaptative pain (acute pain) is the normal process that protects the body from injury; maladaptive pain (chronic pain) is the change to nociceptive sensory systems that may occur when tissue injury or inflammation occurs, and sensitivity of the injured area is heightened.[7] The progression from adaptive to maladaptive pain (wind-up) can be viewed as a spectrum of activity-dependent progressive increases in response of neurons to nociceptor stimuli.[7] *Peripheral sensitization* results when neurotransmitters and chemical mediators released by damaged cells either directly activate the nociceptor or sensitize the nerve terminals[4]; this can result in long-lasting, functional changes to peripheral nociceptors that can lead to hypersensitivity with later stimulation.[3,4] *Central sensitization* occurs when intense nociception input into the spinal cord and brain is sustained beyond the initiating stimulus[3]; this may lead to amplified responsiveness of nociceptive neurons to normal or subthreshold afferent input and enlarging receptor fields to recruit previously quiet afferent fibers into nociceptive transmission.[4,8] Peripheral and central nociceptive sensitization are the result of neuronal plasticity, defined as changes in properties or functions of neurons that outlast the stimulus that caused the change.[8]

The consequence of peripheral and central sensitization of the nociceptive system manifests clinically as hyperalgesia and allodynia. Hyperalgesia is an exaggerated and prolonged response to a noxious stimulus at a lower threshold and can be divided into primary hyperalgesia and secondary hyperalgesia.[3,4] Primary hyperalgesia is increased sensitivity at the area of injury or inflammation, and secondary hyperalgesia is increased sensitivity in uninjured or inflamed tissues in areas around and beyond the primary injured site.[3] Allodynia is pain in response to a low-intensity, nonpainful stimulation such as a light touch on the skin.[3,4] This pain occurs when there is a failure of inhibitory neurons in the spinal cord and cross-talk takes place between low threshold Aβ fibers (nonnoxious fibers responsible for discerning touch) and ascending nociceptive neurons.[5]

Addressing maladaptive pain is commonplace in a rehabilitation setting. The pain management plan should strive to use a multimodal approach, as transmission of pain is complex. Interrupting pain via multiple pathways has been shown to be more effective than relying on a single mechanism.[9,10] The employment of multiple strategies and a coordinated team approach can provide continuous and overlapping pain relief for the patient.

Recognition of Pain

The expression of pain is species-specific and can be influenced by a variety of factors including age, breed, temperament, anxiety, and fear. The goal is to accurately assess, recognize, and alleviate pain in the patient.[11] The physical examination is the primary tool in assessing pain with close monitoring of nonverbal cues (eg, holding breath, lip-licking), but must also include the clinical observation of posture, gait, and behavior.[12] Common behavioral signs include change in posture or body position, change in attitude (aggressive or passive), vocalization, abnormal reaction to touch, reduction in appetite, and alterations in sleep/wake patterns.[6]

Palpation is the most common clinical tool to detect pain but should be correlated with additional assessment tools to improve specificity.[13] Physiologic variables (heart rate, respiration, blood pressure), wound palpation, home videos, gait analysis (force plate and pressure sensitive walkway), and actigraphy (activity monitoring) are all methods to aid in pain recognition.[12] The clinical metrology instruments are also an important component of screening and monitoring for pain and include the Canine Osteoarthritis Staging Tool (COAST), Colorado Acute Pain Scale, Canine Brief Pain Inventory (CBPI), Liverpool Osteoarthritis in Dogs (LOAD), and Glasgow Short Form.[14,15]

Pharmacologic Interventions

Nonsteroidal antiinflammatory drugs

Nonsteroidal antiinflammatory drugs (NSAIDs) are the most used pharmacological intervention in a rehabilitation setting, most often with osteoarthritis patients. These drugs exert their effects on different pathways (**Fig. 1**) of the arachidonic acid cascade.[16] NSAID analgesic and antiinflammatory effects are related to the inhibition of cyclooxygenase (COX) enzyme expression on cell membranes.[16] Cyclooxygenase-1 (COX-1) and COX-2 are key enzymes in prostaglandin production, with COX-2 primarily released after tissue injury, which contributes to inflammation and pain.[16,17] When COX-2 enzymes are inhibited by NSAIDs, the biosynthesis of prostaglandins responsible for the production of inflammatory mediators (endotoxins, cytokines, growth factors) is inhibited.[16,18] Common selective coxib class medications include carprofen, deracoxib, firocoxib, meloxicam, and robenacoxib.[16]

Grapiprant, a piprant class medication, has a different mode of action than the coxib class medications and is considered an EP4 prostaglandin receptor antagonist.[19] Arachidonic acid is converted by COX enzymes into active prostanoid metabolites that have various physiologic functions throughout the body.[16,19] Prostaglandin E_2 (PGE_2) has homeostatic functions as well as being a key mediator of swelling, redness, and pain resulting from PGE_2-mediated sensitization of sensory neurons.[19] When PGE_2 binds to the EP4 receptor, this coupling contributes to pain and inflammation.[16] Grapiprant functions as a potent and highly selective antagonist of PGE_2 to the EP4 receptor site.[16,20]

Adjunct Pain Medications

Acetaminophen acts primarily as an analgesic and antipyretic with weak antiinflammatory effects.[21] It can inhibit prostaglandin E2 synthesis activity in the central nervous system and inhibit central COX receptors, but the exact analgesic mechanisms are unknown and may affect cannabinoid receptors and serotonergic pathways.[22,23] Acetaminophen is well tolerated by dogs but the research is mixed on its efficacy in

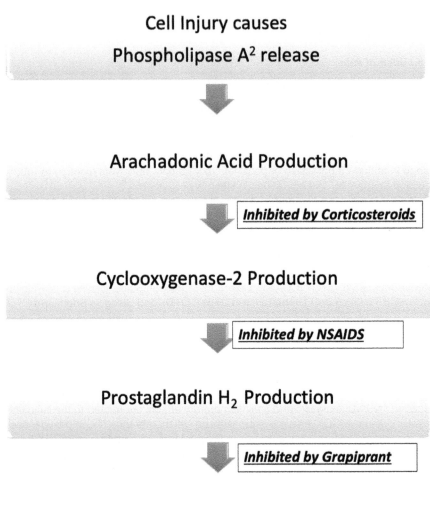

Fig. 1. Arachidonic acid cascade and site of action of various medications.

veterinary medicine.[21,22,24] Acetaminophen is contraindicated in cats due to deficient glucuronidation, which makes them extremely sensitive to toxicity.[16]

Amantadine and ketamine are N-methyl-D-aspartate (NMDA) receptor antagonists.[3] NMDA receptors, located in the spinal cord and brain, are activated with repeat input from afferent nociceptive signals, which can lead to prolonged depolarization and neurobiological changes that prolong inflammatory and neuropathic pain ("wind up").[25] Amantadine as an oral medication or a subanesthetic dose of SQ ketamine can produce antihyperalgesic effects as a treatment of maladaptive pain.[26,27]

Gabapentin has been found to be beneficial in the management of neuropathic pain, as it decreases central sensitization by binding to calcium channels in the dorsal horn of the spinal cord, which prevents release of glutamate into the nociceptive pathways.[28] Gabapentin may also antagonize the NMDA receptor, which can potentially decrease allodynia and hyperalgesia.[29] In human medicine, gabapentin is approved as an adjunct antiepileptic and antihyperalgesic drug; in veterinary medicine it is widely used for chronic pain management.[26]

Tramadol is a central acting synthetic weak opioid agonist and a serotonin and norepinephrine reuptake inhibitor.[26] Tramadol is metabolized into active M1 metabolites that bind to the μ-opioid receptor to produce analgesia; however, it has been shown to be ineffective as a solo analgesic agent for dogs with pain.[30] Tramadol has shown better analgesic efficacy in cats although issues of palatability can make administration difficult.[31,32]

Frunevetmab is a monthly subcutaneous felinized monoclonal antibody injection recently approved for osteoarthritis in cats. It functions to block the receptor-mediated signaling cascade produced by nerve growth factor (NGF).[33] NGF is critical for the developing nervous system in prenatal and early postnatal periods; however, in adults NGF shifts to modulation of nociception and is expressed in areas of injury and inflammation.[34,35]

Intraarticular Interventions

Intraarticular (IA) injections of corticosteroids have been successfully used to improve the comfort and mitigate the pain of osteoarthritic patients.[36] Triamcinolone is a long-acting corticosteroid and is the preferred IA corticosteroid, as it has been shown to not have the detrimental effects on chondrocytes and synoviocytes as other long-acting preparations.[37] Triamcinolone works to reduce the number of inflammatory cell types (lymphocytes, macrophages, and so forth) and inflammatory mediators (interleukin-1 [IL-1β], tumor necrosis factor alpha, COX-2, and so forth) in addition to blocking the production of prostaglandin to provide pain relief.[36] IA triamcinolone is frequently paired with hyaluronic acid (HA) for visco\ementation of the joint and a multimodal approach to pain relief. HA is a high molecular glycosaminoglycan that is present in synovial fluid and provides lubrication and viscoelasticity to decrease degradation in joints and maintain joint homeostasis.[36,38] In addition, HA mitigates the activities of proinflammatory mediators, mitigates the effect of pronociceptive neuropeptides, and decreases nerve impulses and sensitivity related to osteoarthritis pain.[39]

Regenerative therapeutics most used in rehabilitation medicine are mesenchymal stem cells (MSCs), platelet rich plasma (PRP), autologous conditioned serum (ACS), and autologous protein solution (APS). MSCs are progenitor cells and are typically harvested from adipose tissue or bone marrow. MSCs are considered to be hypoimmunogenic, and pain relief is achieved mainly via the ability to downregulate proinflammatory cytokines with paracrine effects of the patient's immune response.[40,41] PRP is an enriched plasma containing a variety of growth factors that are powerful chemoattractors and mitogens that enhance cell proliferation, cell migration, angiogenesis, and support extracellular matrix production.[42,43] PRP is frequently used solo but can be combined with MSCs.[44] ACS and APS are blood-derived orthobiologics that produce hemoderivatives with high concentrations of IL-1 receptor antagonist (IL-1Ra).[45] IL-1Ra is an antiinflammatory protein that competes for the same receptor as the proinflammatory IL-1β.[45] When IL-1Ra binds to its receptor a proinflammatory pathway is inhibited, thereby mitigating pain.[46]

Intraarticular nuclear medicine comes in the form of a Tin-117m (^{117m}Sn) colloid radiosynoviorthesis (RSO) device. RSO is an emerging therapy targeting the synovial membrane in osteoarthritic joints. Normal synovium is devoid of inflammatory cells; however, when the joint has synovitis, this inflammatory process is the driver of osteoarthritic changes, leading to pain and decreased mobility for the patient.[47] RSO mitigates the synovitis with low-energy ionizing radiation emitted by a radionuclide that penetrates the synovial membrane to eliminate inflamed synoviocytes and decrease pain and inflammation.[48] The RSO agent is given as an outpatient procedure under light sedation, is well tolerated, and has shown no adverse effects on the joint.[49]

Nonpharmacologic Interventions

Manual therapy

Manual therapy is broadly defined as using hands-on techniques with a therapeutic intent to improve tissue extensibility; increase range of motion; encourage relaxation; mobilize soft tissue; modulate pain; and decrease swelling, inflammation, and restriction.[50] Most evidence comes from human studies and shows manual therapy to be a primary and effective method to relieve musculoskeletal pain and is generally well tolerated by patients.[51] Manual therapy can include low-velocity mobilizations (joint mobilization, passive range of motion) and soft tissue techniques (massage, trigger point therapy, stretching) to diminish pain.[51] Precise, targeted manual techniques can decrease myalgia, edema, and ischemia in injured tissues, thereby improving comfort at the local level (peripheral sensitization) and spinal cord level (central sensitization).[50]

Therapeutic exercises

Therapeutic exercise in the form of aerobic conditioning, flexibility training, and muscle strengthening combined with the appropriate intensity, frequency, and duration is a key element of nonpharmacologic pain relief. Exercise frequently combined with manual techniques has been shown to improve outcomes for patients with pain and limited mobility.[51] Exercise performed in the water (walking, swimming) can significantly reduce weight-bearing stress and discomfort on joints.[52] Buoyancy allows for exercise that may be potentially painful outside of water to be completed more comfortably in an underwater treadmill or pool.[52] Hydrostatic pressure and increased temperature can also lead to increased sensory input and aid in pain relief during exercise.[52] A multimodal exercise program can reduce pain scores and not only provide relief but also allow for flexibility and customization for activities with the ability of progression with patient improvement.[53]

Cryotherapy

Cryotherapy is the therapeutic application of cold and is usually applied in a rehabilitation setting via cold packs, cold compression units, or vapocoolant spray to mitigate acute inflammation and pain.[54] The primary objective of cryotherapy is to decrease the metabolic rate of injured tissue by decreasing tissue temperature.[55] The mechanism of pain relief can be due to a combination of lower sensory and motor nerve conduction velocities, vasoconstriction, and overstimulation of cold receptors blocking transmission of nociception to higher centers.[55] In addition, cold reduces inflammatory mediators and downregulates muscle excitability to decrease muscle spasm.[55,56]

Superficial heat

The application of a superficial heat source is to raise the local tissue temperature to relieve pain, relax muscle spasm, increase local blood supply, and increase soft tissue extensibility.[56] Superficial heat can modulate pain at the local level and via the central nervous system. Activation of peripheral thermoreceptors initiates signals to modulate nociception with the analgesic effects partially mediated by the transient receptor potential vanilloid 1 (TRPV1) receptor.[57] TRPV1 receptors facilitate neural transduction of heat and processing of nociceptive pain.[56] Activation of these receptors in the brain is thought to regulate antinociceptive pathways.[57] Superficial heat also decreases the nerve firing rate of α-motor neurons that contributes to improved muscle relaxation and decreased muscle tonicity, resulting in lessening muscle spasms and musculoskeletal pain.[57] At the local level, superficial heat causes vasodilation, increases blood and lymph flow, and improves reabsorption of edema, which helps remove tissue metabolites and increases tissue oxygenation and metabolic rate.[56] Heat can be applied in a variety of ways. Hot packs/heating pads are the most common method with 1 to 2 cm depth of penetration; however, a therapeutic ultrasound can also be used for deeper penetration of up to 5 cm.[56]

Photobiomodulation

Photobiomodulation therapy (PBMT) is the clinical use of red/near infrared light to stimulate healing, decrease inflammation, and ameliorate pain.[58,59] PBMT uses photons at varying wavelengths and nonthermal irradiance to influence biological activity at the cellular level of gene expression;[60] this results in the synthesis of antiapoptotic proteins and antioxidant enzymes, promotion of cell proliferation and migration, and antiinflammatory signaling.[58,60] Pain relief specifically may be the result of increased serotonin, β-endorphin, and nitric oxide levels; decreased bradykinins and prostaglandin synthesis; normalization of ion channels; and improved axonal sprouting and nerve cell regeneration.[61]

Transcutaneous electrical nerve stimulation

Transcutaneous electrical nerve stimulation (TENS) is the application of low-voltage electrical impulses via electrode on the skin at varying frequencies, amplitudes, and waveforms for pain relief.[62] Both peripheral and central nervous systems are involved in the analgesic action of TENS.[63] Via the gate theory of pain control, electrical currents trigger large cutaneous Aβ fibers to activate inhibitory neurons in the dorsal horn of the spinal cord to block transmission of the pain impulses.[62] In addition, there is a release of endogenous opioids and suppression of inflammatory cytokines, which can reduce central sensitization and hyperalgesia.[56,63]

Pulse electromagnetic field therapy

Pulse electromagnetic field (PEMF) is a noninvasive, nonthermal treatment that produces a small electrical field within the target tissues to provide pain relief via complex biophysical and cellular mechanisms.[64] Increased calcium ion signaling and triggering of the calcium calmodulin/constitutive nitric oxide synthase/nitric oxide cascade leads to downstream signaling pathways that reduce the production of proinflammatory factors.[64,65] A significant reduction of pain and opioid use has been demonstrated in both human and veterinary randomized controlled studies when PEMF is used postoperatively.[66,67]

Extracorporeal shockwave therapy

Extracorporeal shockwave therapy (ESWT) is the application of a sonic pulse (acoustic pressure or sound wave) to targeted tissues to reduce pain and inflammation of various musculoskeletal injuries.[68] Although a definitive mechanism of action has not been identified, ESWT has shown to reduce pain in both human and veterinary studies.[69–71] ESWT may ameliorate pain by promoting neovascularization, reducing inflammatory cytokines, altering substance P, and decreasing sensory nerve conduction velocity.[70]

SUMMARY

Pain management is a primary focus and an integral part of every veterinary rehabilitation practice. Evidence-based pain management protocols will use both pharmacologic and nonpharmacologic tools to create a customized, safe, and effective treatment plan. A multimodal, patient-centered approach will allow for the best outcomes for pain relief and improved quality of life.

CLINICS CARE POINTS

- The recognition of pain and a thorough assessment of the patient is essential in formulating a treatment plan for the painful patient.
- Understanding the physiology and pathophysiology of pain is a key element in pain management.
- It is critical to have a thorough understanding of the mode of action of pharmacologic and nonpharmacologic methods of pain mitigation.
- A multimodal approach for pain management will improve patient outcomes.

DISCLOSURE

The author has nothing to disclose.

REFERENCES

1. Molony V, Kent JE. Assessment of acute pain in farm animals using behavioral and physiological measurements. J Anim Sci 1997;75:266–72.
2. Morton CM, Reid J, Scott EM, et al. Application of a scaling model to establish and validate an interval level pain scale for assessment of acute pain in dogs. Am J Vet Res 2005;66:2154–66.
3. Wiese AJ, yaksh TL. Nociception and pain mechanisms. In: Gaynor JS, Muir WW, editors. Handbook of veterinary pain management. Third edition. St. Louis, Missouri: Elsevier; 2015. p. 10–41.
4. McKune CM, Murrell JC, Nolan AM, et al. Nocieption and pain. In: Grimm KA, Lamont LA, Tranquilli WJ, et al, editors. Veterinary anesthesia and analgesia. Fifth edition. Ames, Iowa: Wiley Blackwell; 2015. p. 584–623.
5. Self I, Grubb, T. Physiology of Pain. In: Self I. British Small Animal Veterinary Veterinary Association Guide to Pain Management in Small Animal Practice: British Small Animal Veterinary Association, Gloucester (England): 2019.p. 3-13.
6. Mathews K, Kronen PW, Lascelles D, et al. Guidelines for recognition, assessment and treatment of pain: WSAVA Global Pain Council members and co-authors of this document. J Small Anim Pract 2014;55:E10–68.
7. Fox SM, Downing R. Rehabilitating the painful patient: pain management in physical rehabilitation. In: Millis DL, Levine D, editors. Canine rehabilitation and physical therapy. Second edition. Philadelphia, PA: Elsevier; 2014. p. 243–53.
8. Sandkuhler J. Spinal cord plasticity and pain. In: McMahon SB, editor. Wall and Melzack's textbook of pain. 6th ed. Philadelphia, PA: Elsevier/Saunders; 2013. p. 94–110.
9. Slingsby LS, Waterman-Pearson AE. Analgesic effects in dogs of carprofen and pethidine together compared with the effects of either drug alone. Vet Rec 2001; 148:441–4.

10. Grzanna MW, Secor EJ, Fortuno LV, et al. Anti-inflammatory effect of carprofen is enhanced by avocado/soybean unsaponifiables, glucosamine and chondroitin sulfate combination in chondrocyte microcarrier spinner culture. Cartilage 2020;11:108–16.

11. Morton DB, Griffiths PH. Guidelines on the recognition of pain, distress and discomfort in experimental animals and an hypothesis for assessment. Vet Rec 1985;116:431–6.

12. Gruen ME, Lascelles BDX, Colleran E, et al. 2022 AAHA pain management guidelines for dogs and cats. J Am Anim Hosp Assoc 2022;58:55–76.

13. Carobbi B, Ness MG. Preliminary study evaluating tests used to diagnose canine cranial cruciate ligament failure. J Small Anim Pract 2009;50:224–6.

14. Epstein M, Kuehn NF, Landsberg G, et al. AAHA senior care guidelines for dogs and cats. J Am Anim Hosp Assoc 2005;41:81–91.

15. Cachon T, Frykman O, Innes JF, et al. Face validity of a proposed tool for staging canine osteoarthritis: canine osteoarthritis staging tool (COAST). Vet J 2018; 235:1–8.

16. Monteiro B, Steagall PV. Antiinflammatory drugs. Vet Clin North Am Small Anim Pract 2019;49:993–1011.

17. Enthoven WT, Roelofs PD, Deyo RA, et al. Non-steroidal anti-inflammatory drugs for chronic low back pain. Cochrane Database Syst Rev 2016;2:Cd012087.

18. Lees P, Landoni MF, Giraudel J, et al. Pharmacodynamics and pharmacokinetics of nonsteroidal anti-inflammatory drugs in species of veterinary interest. J Vet Pharmacol Ther 2004;27:479–90.

19. Kirkby Shaw K, Rausch-Derra LC, Rhodes L. Grapiprant: an EP4 prostaglandin receptor antagonist and novel therapy for pain and inflammation. Vet Med Sci 2016;2:3–9.

20. Rausch-Derra L, Huebner M, Wofford J, et al. A Prospective, randomized, masked, placebo-controlled multisite clinical study of grapiprant, an ep4 prostaglandin receptor antagonist (PRA), in dogs with osteoarthritis. J Vet Intern Med 2016;30:756–63.

21. Hernández-Avalos I, Valverde A, Ibancovichi-Camarillo JA, et al. Clinical evaluation of postoperative analgesia, cardiorespiratory parameters and changes in liver and renal function tests of paracetamol compared to meloxicam and carprofen in dogs undergoing ovariohysterectomy. PLoS One 2020;15:e0223697.

22. Leung J, Beths T, Carter JE, et al. Intravenous acetaminophen does not provide adequate postoperative analgesia in dogs following ovariohysterectomy. Animals (Basel) 2021,1–10.

23. Chandrasekharan NV, Dai H, Roos KL, et al. COX-3, a cyclooxygenase-1 variant inhibited by acetaminophen and other analgesic/antipyretic drugs: cloning, structure, and expression. Proc Natl Acad Sci U S A 2002;99:13926–31.

24. KuKanich B. Pharmacokinetics and pharmacodynamics of oral acetaminophen in combination with codeine in healthy greyhound dogs. J Vet Pharmacol Ther 2016;39:514–7.

25. Lascelles BD, Gaynor JS, Smith ES, et al. Amantadine in a multimodal analgesic regimen for alleviation of refractory osteoarthritis pain in dogs. J Vet Intern Med 2008;22:53–9.

26. Ruel HLM, Steagall PV. Adjuvant analgesics in acute pain management. Vet Clin North Am Small Anim Pract 2019;49:1127–41.

27. Silva E, Schumacher J, Passler T. Castration of dogs using local anesthesia after sedating with xylazine and subanesthetic doses of ketamine. Front Vet Sci 2019; 6:478.

28. Davis L, Hellyer P, Downing R, et al. Retrospective study of 240 dogs receiving gabapentin for chronic pain relief. J Vet Med Res 2020;7(4):1194.

29. Johnson BA, Aarnes TK, Wanstrath AW, et al. Effect of oral administration of gabapentin on the minimum alveolar concentration of isoflurane in dogs. Am J Vet Res 2019;80:1007–9.

30. Budsberg SC, Torres BT, Kleine SA, et al. Lack of effectiveness of tramadol hydrochloride for the treatment of pain and joint dysfunction in dogs with chronic osteoarthritis. J Am Vet Med Assoc 2018;252:427–32.

31. Guedes AGP, Meadows JM, Pypendop BH, et al. Evaluation of tramadol for treatment of osteoarthritis in geriatric cats. J Am Vet Medl Assoc 2018;252:565–71.

32. Monteiro BP, Klinck MP, Moreau M, et al. Analgesic efficacy of tramadol in cats with naturally occurring osteoarthritis. PLoS One 2017;12:e0175565.

33. Walters RR, Boucher JF, De Toni F. Pharmacokinetics and immunogenicity of frunevetmab in osteoarthritic cats following intravenous and subcutaneous administration. Front Vet Sci 2021;8:687448.

34. Enomoto M, Mantyh PW, Murrell J, et al. Anti-nerve growth factor monoclonal antibodies for the control of pain in dogs and cats. Vet Rec 2019;184:23.

35. Gearing DP, Huebner M, Virtue ER, et al. In Vitro and In Vivo characterization of a fully felinized therapeutic anti-nerve growth factor monoclonal antibody for the treatment of pain in cats. J Vet Intern Med 2016;30:1129–37.

36. Alves JC, Santos A, Jorge P, et al. A pilot study on the efficacy of a single intra-articular administration of triamcinolone acetonide, hyaluronan, and a combination of both for clinical management of osteoarthritis in police working dogs. Front Vet Sci 2020;7:512523.

37. Sherman SL, Khazai RS, James CH, et al. In Vitro toxicity of local anesthetics and corticosteroids on chondrocyte and synoviocyte viability and metabolism. Cartilage 2015;6:233–40.

38. Kilborne AH, Hussein H, Bertone AL. Effects of hyaluronan alone or in combination with chondroitin sulfate and N-acetyl-d-glucosamine on lipopolysaccharide challenge-exposed equine fibroblast-like synovial cells. Am J Vet Res 2017;78:579–88.

39. Gupta RC, Lall R, Srivastava A, et al. Hyaluronic acid: molecular mechanisms and therapeutic trajectory. Front Vet Sci 2019;6:192.

40. Pye C, Bruniges N, Peffers M, et al. Advances in the pharmaceutical treatment options for canine osteoarthritis. J Small Anim Pract 2022;63:721–38.

41. Voga M, Adamic N, Vengust M, et al. Stem cells in veterinary medicine-current state and treatment options. Front Vet Sci 2020;7:278.

42. Pandey S, Hickey DU, Drum M, et al. Platelet-rich plasma affects the proliferation of canine bone marrow-derived mesenchymal stromal cells in vitro. BMC (Biomed Chromatogr) 2019;15:269.

43. Sample SJ, Racette MA, Hans EC, et al. Use of a platelet-rich plasma-collagen scaffold as a bioenhanced repair treatment for management of partial cruciate ligament rupture in dogs. PLoS One 2018;13:e0197204.

44. Canapp SO Jr, Leasure CS, Cox C, et al. Partial cranial cruciate ligament tears treated with stem cell and platelet-rich plasma combination therapy in 36 dogs: a retrospective study. Front Vet Sci 2016;3:112.

45. Camargo Garbin L, Morris MJ. A comparative review of autologous conditioned serum and autologous protein solution for treatment of osteoarthritis in horses. Front Vet Sci 2021;8:602978.

46. Wanstrath AW, Hettlich BF, Su L, et al. Evaluation of a single intra-articular injection of autologous protein solution for treatment of osteoarthritis in a canine population. Vet Surg 2016;45:764–74.

47. Donecker J, Lattimer JC, Gaschen L, et al. Safety and clinical response following a repeat intraarticular injection of Tin-117m ((117m)Sn) colloid in dogs with elbow osteoarthritis. Vet Med (Auckl) 2021;12:325–35.

48. Donecker J, Fabiani M, Gaschen L, et al. Treatment response in dogs with naturally occurring grade 3 elbow osteoarthritis following intra-articular injection of 117mSn (tin) colloid. PLoS One 2021;16:e0254613.

49. Lattimer JC, Selting KA, Lunceford JM, et al. Intraarticular injection of a Tin-117 m radiosynoviorthesis agent in normal canine elbows causes no adverse effects. Vet Radiol Ultrasound 2019;60:567–74.

50. Lederman E. Manual therapy in the tissue dimension. In: Wolfaard S, editor. The science and practice of manual therapy. 2nd ed. Edinburgh ; New York: Elsevier/Churchill Livingstone; 2005. p. 9–12.

51. Hidalgo B, Hall T, Bossert J, et al. The efficacy of manual therapy and exercise for treating non-specific neck pain: A systematic review. J Back Musculoskeletal Rehabil 2017;30:1149–69.

52. Dias JM, Cisneros L, Dias R, et al. Hydrotherapy improves pain and function in older women with knee osteoarthritis: a randomized controlled trial. Braz J Phys Ther 2017;21:449–56.

53. Drum MG, Marcellin-Little DJ, Davis MS. Principles and applications of therapeutic exercises for small animals. Vet Clin North Am Small Anim Pract 2015;45: 73–90.

54. Hanks J, Levine D, Bockstahler B. Physical agent modalities in physical therapy and rehabilitation of small animals. Vet Clin North Am Small Anim Pract 2015;45: 29–44.

55. Drygas KA, McClure SR, Goring RL, et al. Effect of cold compression therapy on postoperative pain, swelling, range of motion, and lameness after tibial plateau leveling osteotomy in dogs. J Am Vet Med Assoc 2011;238:1284–91.

56. Niebaum K. Rehabilitation physical modalities. In: Zink C, VanDyke JB, editors. Canine sports medicine and rehabilitation. Ames (Iowa): Wiley Blackwell; 2013. p. 115–31.

57. Freiwald J, Magni A, Fanlo-Mazas P, et al. A role for superficial heat therapy in the management of non-specific, mild-to-moderate low back pain in current clinical practice: a narrative review. Life 2021;11:1–13.

58. Looney AL, Huntingford JL, Blaeser LL, et al. A randomized blind placebo-controlled trial investigating the effects of photobiomodulation therapy (PBMT) on canine elbow osteoarthritis. Can Vet J 2018;59:959–66.

59. Alves JC, Santos A, Jorge P, et al. A randomized double-blinded controlled trial on the effects of photobiomodulation therapy in dogs with osteoarthritis. Am J Vet Res 2022;83:1–8.

60. Marchegiani A, Spaterna A, Cerquetella M. Current applications and future perspectives of fluorescence light energy biomodulation in veterinary medicine. Vet Sci 2021;8:1–11.

61. Pryor B, Millis DL. Therapeutic laser in veterinary medicine. Vet Clin North Am Small Anim Pract 2015;45:45–56.

62. Flaherty MJ. Rehabilitation therapy in perioperative pain management. Vet Clin North Am Small Anim Pract 2019;49:1143–56.

63. Zhu Y, Feng Y, Peng L. Effect of transcutaneous electrical nerve stimulation for pain control after total knee arthroplasty: a systematic review and meta-analysis. J Rehabil Med 2017;49:700–4.
64. Gaynor JS, Hagberg S, Gurfein BT. Veterinary applications of pulsed electromagnetic field therapy. Res Vet Sci 2018;119:1–8.
65. Zidan N, Fenn J, Griffith E, et al. The effect of electromagnetic fields on postoperative pain and locomotor recovery in dogs with acute, severe thoracolumbar intervertebral disc extrusion: a randomized placebo-controlled, prospective clinical trial. J Neurotrauma 2018;35:1726–36.
66. Alvarez LX, McCue J, Lam NK, et al. Effect of targeted pulsed electromagnetic field therapy on canine postoperative hemilaminectomy: a double-blind, randomized, placebo-controlled clinical trial. J Am Anim Hosp Assoc 2019;55:83–91.
67. Rohde C, Chiang A, Adipoju O, et al. Effects of pulsed electromagnetic fields on interleukin-1 beta and postoperative pain: a double-blind, placebo-controlled, pilot study in breast reduction patients. Plast Reconstr Surg 2010;125:1620–9.
68. Kieves NR, MacKay CS, Adducci K, et al. High energy focused shock wave therapy accelerates bone healing. A blinded, prospective, randomized canine clinical trial. Vet Comp Orthop Traumatol 2015;28:425–32.
69. Zhong Z, Liu B, Liu G, et al. A randomized controlled trial on the effects of low-dose extracorporeal shockwave therapy in patients with knee osteoarthritis. Arch Phys Med Rehabil 2019;100:1695–702.
70. Barnes K, Faludi A, Takawira C, et al. Extracorporeal shock wave therapy improves short-term limb use after canine tibial plateau leveling osteotomy. Vet Surg 2019;48:1382–90.
71. An S, Li J, Xie W, et al. Extracorporeal shockwave treatment in knee osteoarthritis: therapeutic effects and possible mechanism. Biosci Rep 2020;40:1–8.

Select Manual Assessment Techniques and Clinical Reasoning Skills Used in Canine Physical Rehabilitation Before Engaging in Manual Therapy Treatment

Laurie Edge-Hughes, BScPT, MAnimSt, CCRT, CAFCI[a],*,
Amy Lee Kramer, DPT, CCRT[b], Ria Acciani, MPT, CCRP[c]

KEYWORDS

- Clinical reasoning • Manual therapy • Physical therapy • Chiropractic • Osteopathy
- Functional diagnosis • Canine rehabilitation • Physical examination

KEY POINTS

- Clinical reasoning skills are fundamental in canine physical rehabilitation as a method of making sense of all data collected during an examination and formulating a functional diagnosis.
- Observation skills allow analysis of posture and movement patterns that further guide the direction of the physical examination.
- Manual assessment skills consider selective tissue tension techniques, end feels, and palpation findings.
- The culmination of clinical reasoning, observations, and manual assessment techniques can serve to direct the treatment plan including what, where, when, and how manual therapy should be performed to help achieve the rehabilitation goals.

INTRODUCTION

Manual therapy is a cornerstone of treatment in physical therapy and canine physical rehabilitation. Its effectiveness has been validated and mechanisms of action expanded upon within the last decade.[1,2] Of equal importance, however, is the determination of

[a] The Canine Fitness Centre Ltd, 4515 Manhattan Road. Southeast, Calgary, AB T2G 4B3, Canada; [b] Beach Animal Rehabilitation Center, 18837 Hawthorne Boulevard, Torrance, CA 90504, USA; [c] Advanced Canine Rehabilitation Center, 166 Mountainview Road, Warren, NJ 07059, USA
* Corresponding author.
E-mail address: Laurie@caninefitness.com

Vet Clin Small Anim 53 (2023) 743–756
https://doi.org/10.1016/j.cvsm.2023.02.007
0195-5616/23/© 2023 Elsevier Inc. All rights reserved.

when manual therapy techniques should be used to achieve a desired goal or outcome. Current veterinary literature is lacking in regards to the manual assessment techniques that guide manual therapy interventions.

First, the goals of the animal owner need to be established to ensure they are realistic. The next step is to assess the patient through use of clinical reasoning skills and a comprehensive masterful manual assessment. This article will discuss how to use clinical reasoning skills and a select grouping of assessment techniques that will help the clinician arrive at a functional diagnosis in order to guide a treatment plan that includes manual therapies.

Clinical Reasoning

Clinical reasoning has been defined as a process in which the clinician interacts with the patient (or in the veterinary setting, the owner), and structures meaning, goals and health management strategies based on scientific evidence, clinical data, patient/ owner choices and professional judgment and knowledge.[1]

The process of clinical reasoning is interactive and dynamic and can lead to a functional diagnosis, differential diagnoses, and/or a clinical hypothesis. The aim is to identify all causal and correlative factors and subsequently prioritize treatment approaches. This process is not an alternative to traditional diagnostics but it is helpful in determining what, if any, further diagnostics are indicated. Additionally, consideration needs to be given to the fact that rarely in animal rehabilitation is there a singular diagnosis for all that is affecting the animal patient. There are often additional or secondary dysfunctions related to, causal to, or affected by the primary "diagnosis," which are likely to require additional remediation efforts.

The aim of the functional diagnosis is to diagnose movement system impairments to guide intervention for health optimization such that the disability can be minimized.[3] The key diagnostic questions addressed are as follows: (1) What are the impairments, their nature and source? (2) Which impairments are related to the patient's functional limitation? (3) Which among these can be remedied by intervention? (4) What is the influence of the contextual (environment and individual) factor of a patient in his function? (5) Can the contextual factors be changed or remedied to maximize performance? (6) What is the diagnostic label? Although the medical diagnosis might identify the structure at the root of the issue, it is insufficient to guide a comprehensive rehabilitation strategy. As such rehabilitation practitioners use their own functional diagnoses to proceed with manual therapies or other treatments.

In animal rehabilitation, the process of clinical reasoning should consider signalment, breed predisposition, and progression of clinical signs over time with or without treatment. Bayesian probability is an interpretation of the concept of probability, in which, instead of frequency or propensity of some phenomenon, probability is interpreted as a reasonable expectation representing a state of knowledge or as quantification of a personal belief.[4] A recent article reinvigorated the concept of Bayesian clinical reasoning in application to the diagnosis of an intervertebral disc extrusion in a chondrodystrophic dog.[5] "Bayesian clinical reasoning is a way of taking into account the known pretest probability of a disorder (based on a mix of published reviews, studies and case reports, and expert opinion), and using this information to interpret the probability of that disorder following the results of a diagnostic test."[5] For example, acute pancreatitis is known to present with vague, nonspecific signs including pain alone in the cranial abdominal region, which can commonly be misdiagnosed in cases of intervertebral disc extrusion, and vice versa.[6] However, clinical experience tells us that a 5-year-old dachshund will most likely have a disc extrusion, whereas a middle-aged miniature schnauzer is more likely to have pancreatitis.

Clinical progression, response to treatment, combined with signalment can almost be considered a "test," which will not only meet many of the criteria previously described but also lead to many dogs recovering without the requirement for further testing.[5]

A variety of components are considered when a practitioner engages in clinical reasoning as part of the assessment process. **Table 1** has been modified to fit the canine model and addresses contexts and metaskills of clinical reasoning.[7]

The skills required to guide orthopedic manual physical therapy have been established by consensus.[8] They include the ability to accurately and efficiently select inquiry strategies based on early recognition and correct interpretation of relevant clinical cues; the ability to reflect and self-evaluate in managing patients; knowledge of the specific special tests/screening tests for the safe practice of orthopedic manual therapy; creativity and innovation in the application of knowledge of orthopedic manual physical therapy; knowledge of effectiveness, risks, and efficacy of orthopedic manual therapy interventions; knowledge of the specific diagnostic and evaluative qualities of assessment tools; knowledge of prognostic, risk, and predictive factors of relevant problems and their impact on orthopedic manual therapy management strategies; the ability to identify the nature and extent of patient's functional abilities, pain, and multidimensional needs; the ability to determine which assessment and intervention tools are most appropriate; the ability to interpret outcomes of assessment and interventions; and the ability to accurately predict expected changes and progress toward realistic outcomes. The skilled canine manual therapy practitioner needs to be equally cognizant and trained in these areas.

For the purpose of this publication, the authors will focus on visual assessment of gait and posture, and the manual assessment techniques of selective tissue tension (STT), end feels, and palpation because they factor into clinical reasoning processes and the formation of a functional diagnosis. The culmination of all components is what effectively guides treatment through manual therapy interventions.

Observation of Movement and Posture

Jiandani and Mhatre (2018) state that the aim of a physical therapy diagnosis or functional diagnosis is to diagnose movement system impairments to guide intervention

---

Table 1
Contexts and metaskills of clinical reasoning in canine rehabilitation

Contexts

Practitioner	Patient
• Practice knowledge	• Preexisting medical conditions/comorbidities
• Practice experience	• Breed conformation
• Values and beliefs	• Progression of clinical signs
• Own professional practice	(with or without treatment)
Owner	• Job
• Home environment	
• Goals of patient	

Metaskills

- Knowledge of animal behavior
- Understanding of canine body language
- Understanding of breed disposition
- Analytic skills and pattern recognition

Adapted from: Higgs J, Jones M. Clinical reasoning in the health professions. In: Higgs J, Jones M, Loftus S, et al., editors. Clinical reasoning in the health professions. Edinburgh: Butterworth Heinemann; 2008. p. 24.

for health optimization such that the disability can be minimized.[3] As such, the observational portion of the assessment detects movement impairments associated with the underlying pathology, which can then be further investigated during the subjective history and manual evaluation.

Observational skills are an expertise unto themselves. Via observation of informal movements about the examination room as well as a formal gait analysis, the rehab practitioner takes note not only of lameness or off-loading of a limb but also of head position, tail position, thoracic and pelvic limb placement, structure, asymmetries, muscling, stride length, weight-bearing, spinal position and movement, and hair anomalies, and so forth. Even at this early stage, the experienced practitioner can start formulating a plan for their physical examination.

These same observations will take place as you look at posture in standing, sitting, and lying. Transitions will be equally important to note as well, along with 3-legged standing for balance and strength. One should then formally look for conformational abnormalities, head position, thoracic and pelvic limb placement, structure, asymmetries, muscling, weight distribution, and hair anomalies. Additionally, spinal position, such as sway, roaching, curvature; pelvic position; and tail position should be noticed. It is beyond the scope of this article to identify every possible gait deviation but to highlight selected observations seen during gait and posture with certain diagnosis.

Posture and Balance

The practitioner should have knowledge of typical weight-bearing patterns in normal dogs and those with orthopedic or neurological conditions. This will provide information that may be valuable in the rehabilitation of the canine patient. Posture is generally evaluated first, and any deviations from normal can be observed and then further confirmed in movement analysis. Conformation is also a factor to consider when evaluating posture. Conformational faults alone can predispose structures to abnormal stresses that could result in injury.[9]

For example, a dog may be shifting its weight off the affected limb, and one would observe that compensations may occur in a contralateral limb or diagonal limb. Further observation may reveal that the paw of a compensating limb may be splayed due to increased weight-bearing and a spinal sway away from the affected limb with thoracic spine roaching (if the lame limb is the forelimb) or lumbar/pelvic flexion (if the affected limb is in the rear). Static balance should also be a part of the postural examination (ie, 3-legged stand, and transitional movements.)

Movement Analysis

Mondino and colleagues[10] (2022) and Lasceles and colleagues[11] (2006) determined that pressure-sensitive walkway systems and force plates are a reliable tool to evaluate gait in dogs. However, many clinics do not have these types of gait analysis tools. Therefore, observational skills and clinical reasoning direct the practitioner toward the areas requiring further physical evaluation.

When observing gait, it is best to use symmetric gaits, such as the walk and trot. Lameness scores can be used as an assessment tool within the clinic.[9,12] However, lameness scores do not describe gait abnormalities. Key factors to observe are stride length, stance phase, weight-bearing, thoracic and pelvic limb placement and carriage, head position, ataxia, spinal position, or asymmetries. It has been noted that severe lesions may cause overt lameness, whereas, a lesser lesion may produce a weight-bearing lameness or gait alteration.[9] Both scenarios cause the dog to alter their gait subsequently causing compensatory weight shifts that affect other parts of the quadruped's body. For example, if the right elbow is involved the contralateral limb will be impacted due to the increased weight-bearing on that limb. This shift in weight then can affect the lower cervical spine, upper thoracic spine, left shoulder and the diagonal pelvic limb, which then can affect the lumbar spine, and pelvis depending on the chronicity of the injury.

Cranial Cruciate Ligament Disease

After cranial cruciate ligament rupture (CCLR), peak vertical force may be only 50% of normal at a walk, and dogs may be non–weight-bearing at a trot.[13] Initially, weight-bearing is increased onto the contralateral rear limb,[13,14] likely from the compensation of the affected limb. It has been found in many kinematic studies that dogs with CCLR demonstrate altered movement in the coxofemoral, femorotibial, and tarsal joints.[14–16] The femorotibial joint angle in the cruciate-deficient state was more flexed throughout the stance and early swing phase of stride and failed to extend fully in the late stance, when limb propulsion is typically developed. The coxofemoral joints in contrast were extended more during the stance phase, perhaps due to compensatory changes.[12] This pattern of CCLR pathological gait provides valuable objective information that can guide the physical examination and subsequent rehabilitation treatment.

Hip Dysplasia

Clinical observations of dogs with hip dysplasia include exercise intolerance, stiffness on rising, bunny hopping, a narrow-based stance, a side-to-side or waddle-like gait, circumduction, shuffling feet, and signs of joint pain with passive range of motion (PROM) and lameness. The degree of lameness is variable and may be mild or severe, and some affected dogs may not be lame.[17] Poy and colleagues[17] (2000) found that dogs with hip dysplasia had a greater degree of coxofemoral joint adduction and range of abduction-adduction and greater lateral pelvic movement. These findings were derived through kinematic studies; however, visual observation of the same can be noted in a clinical examination. Postural deviations commonly include increased weight-bearing onto the contralateral rear and diagonal thoracic limb, narrow-based stance in the rear (affected limb may be slightly held cranially and adducted) and increased lumbar flexion.

Elbow Osteoarthritis

Elbow osteoarthritis is a deterioration of the joint usually secondary to joint incongruity, instability, or some other disruption of the articular cartilage. Bockstahler and colleagues (2009) showed that during posture the load was reduced on the affected limb and increased on the contralateral forelimb and the diagonal hind limb, which resulted in a more balanced weight distribution. During gait analysis, in this same study, the weight redistribution was seen primarily to the contralateral hind limb. These results suggested that forelimb lameness could lead to overload on nonaffected extremities and the vertebral spine.[18] Observing these postural shifts can guide the clinician toward areas that may need further manual evaluation to detect secondary areas of concern.

Intervertebral Disk Disease

Intervertebral disk disease (IVDD) can affect the cervical, thoracic, and lumbar spine. Common presentations in posture and gait can vary depending on the location and severity of the lesion. Neck pain is common in cervical IVDD and may often be the only sign.[9] In these cases, head carriage is low during stance and gait, and there may be short "stutter" stepping gait in the thoracic limbs. Thoracolumbar IVDD is the most common form of disc disease, it accounts for 66% to 86% of all cases.[19]

It has been noted that dogs with acute thoracolumbar IVDD managed surgically tend to lean forward during their recovery period.[20] This is likely in response to ongoing pelvic limb weakness and possible lack of or decrease in proprioception. Lumbosacral disc disease or cauda equina syndrome is in general terms describing compression, inflammation, or vascular compromise of the nerve roots of the cauda equina. Presentation in stance commonly reveals a roaching of the caudal spine (**Fig. 1**), weight distribution cranially, and skin lesions (lick granulomas) on the tail, genitals, or extremities.[19] Gait abnormalities can display as rear limb ataxia, lameness due to radiculopathy, pelvic limb knuckling or nail scuffing, lumbar flexion, and abnormal tail carriage.

Keen observation is often the first-assessment tool utilized by the animal rehabilitation practitioner. Information garnered during this part of the assessment can direct the clinician to areas of primary and secondary concern, to be further evaluated and confirmed with manual techniques during the physical examination.

The Physical Examination

Once the history has been noted and posture and gait have been analyzed, the skilled rehab practitioner proceeds with a physical examination. Directing their focus on either the spinal joints or the peripheral joints based on the information garnered and following a systematic approach that helps to guide and direct the specific physical tests required to establish a functional diagnosis (**Fig. 2**). In almost every case, a scan of both the spine and the peripheral joints is conducted in order to rule in or rule out the spine as a source of clinical signs and/or to identify additional structures that could be compounding the clinical picture. It is outside the scope of this article to fully describe each test for each joint. As such, selected testing practices will be described below.

Selective Tissue Tension

Dr James Cyriax originally described a systematic approach to physical assessment that has been internationally taught and adopted by orthopedic manual practitioners in a multitude of medical fields.[21,22] One such testing method is that of STT techniques.

The premise behind STT is that a healthy structure functions painlessly; a faulty structure does not. As such, each tissue from which pain could originate is assessed in turn, and as each structure has a known and separate function, the tissue that

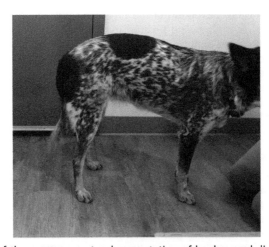

Fig. 1. Example of the common postural presentation of lumbosacral disc disease.

The Scanning Examination

History
Observation
Scanning Exam

Spine - Active and Passive Movements
Peripheral Joints - Active and Passive Range
Myotomes
Neurologic Tests

Educated Guess - Spinal or Peripheral

SPINE	**PERIPHERAL**
Special tests	Active movements
Reflexes	Passive movements
Joint mobility	Special tests
Palpation	Reflexes
	Joint mobility
	Palpation

Are further diagnostics needed?

Fig. 2. A typical scanning examination used to rule in or rule out spinal or peripheral structures as primary or secondary components in the clinical picture.

cannot function without pain is at fault. The mechanism of diagnosis is manually applied tension, and each tissue around a joint is subjected to tension systematically. A standardized STT assessment typically considers active movement, passive movement, and resisted tests.[23] Human studies have demonstrated the Cyriax method of STT testing to provide adequate results, especially for shoulder pathologic conditions where soft tissue structures are common pathologic conditions.[24–26]

During active movements the examiner can observe the following: when and where during each of the movements the onset of pain occurs; whether the movement increases the intensity and quality of the pain; the reaction of the patient to pain; the amount of observable restriction and its nature; the pattern of movement; the rhythm and quality of movement; the movement of associated joints; and the willingness of the patient to move the part.[23] In the canine patient, active movements are best observed while watching a dog gait and observing not only which limb is unsound but also how the animal is moving and compensating. Observation of other tasks or asking questions pertaining to functional abilities (ie, how the animal ascends or descends stairs, sits, gets up from lying, turns, and so forth) may be useful to gather information about active movements and avoidance.

Passive movements provide the animal practitioner with the potential for greater information. PROM should be conducted with the patient as relaxed as possible. Goniometry may be useful for measuring and recording joint deformities and can prove as a useful tool for gauging differences from side to side or alterations of PROM.[23] Goniometry has been studied and found to be reliable in canine applications[27,28]; however, a joint angle number does not convey a functional diagnosis. Of greater diagnostic importance are the examiner observations during passive movement: when and where during each of the movements the pain begins, whether the movement increases the pain, the pattern of limitation of movement, the end feel of movement, the movement of associated joints, and the range of motion available.[23]

Resisted movements are often key to the detection of contractive structures in human patients. This type of movement consists of a strong, static (isometric), voluntary muscle contraction and is used primarily to determine whether the contractile tissue is the tissue at fault, although the nerve supplying the muscle is also tested.[23] The examiner observations during resisted tests would include the following: whether the contraction causes pain and, if it does, the intensity (or quality) of the pain; strength of the contraction; and the type of contraction causing the problem (ie, concentric, eccentric, isometric). Resisted movements are much easier to test in a human patient than an animal patient. However, there may be times when a soft tissue is put on stretch and a practitioner holds the limb in place because the animal fights the hold in an attempt to reposition the limb. Thus, a resisted movement could be evaluated in a canine patient.

Examination example for selective tissue tension testing

When confronted with a canine patient with a suspected supraspinatus tendon pathology, the examiner may find that the animal is demonstrating a lameness when weight-bearing on the affected limb. The canine patient might also lack active shoulder extension during the terminal swing phase of the limb as compared with the contralateral limb. Passive shoulder extension would be full and unremarkable. Shoulder flexion, however, could be painful at end range, where the supraspinatus muscle and tendon are on full stretch. In this scenario, the examiner could pinch a toe with the shoulder in flexion, in an attempt to get the dog to resist his shoulder being held in this position. Pain on resisted contraction of the supraspinatus muscle could lead the examiner toward ruling in supraspinatus as a differential diagnosis. Further testing would ensue whereby other adjacent soft tissue structures where stretched (and resisted), the end feel of the shoulder joint in all ranges would be considered, and palpation of the suspected structures conducted. A culmination of findings could help the practitioner to formulate a working physical diagnosis.

End Feels

End feel to a movement is an important diagnostic indicator. It is the detectable sensation as noted by the examiner's hands at the extreme of a passive movement.[22] The end range of movement is stopped by a variety of structures. Each structure has a different sensation when stressed. Each joint has a different structure that stops motion in any given direction. For example, elbow extension is accompanied by a "Bone to Bone" end feel. This is normal. However, a "bone to bone" end feel would be characterized as abnormal for elbow flexion and could be the result of osteophyte formation and/or osteoarthritis. Those in veterinary medicine that are unfamiliar with the concept of end feels can however likely relate to the physical sensation of testing for cruciate deficiency and noting that a fully torn cranial cruciate ligament presents with a drawer sign that has a distinctly different stopping end feel than that of a fully intact cruciate ligament. **Table 2** is a modification of Cyriax's original listing of end feels.[29] It shows a list of normal and abnormal end feels. It is also possible to have an end feel that is normal for any given joint and movement but that comes on too early in the range.

Utilization of end feels as part of the physical examination has been studied in human medicine. Taken on their own, interrater reliability is variable for determination of an end feel; however, improvements in reliability are noted when consideration is

Table 2
End feels

End Feel	Description	Impression	Normal	Abnormal
Capsular–hard and soft	Produced by capsule or ligament. The end sensation has varying degrees of stretch (depending on the thickness of the capsule or ligaments)	It feels as if further force could tear something	Stifle extension (hard capsular)	Early arthritic changes in a joint can yield a hard capsular end feel before full normal joint range
Bony	An abrupt end to movement, produced by bone on bone approximation	It feels as if further force could break something	Elbow extension	Severe degenerative joint disease affecting ROM in any joint
Elastic	Produced by a muscle-tendon unit. Often occurring with adaptive shortening. A hard feel to the end of movement but with a stretch and elastic recoil effect	It feels as if further force could cause something to snap	Flexion of the tarsus	As with a soft tissue contracture impeding either flexion or extension of any extremity joint
Springy	Produced by the articular surface rebounding from an intra-articular disc or meniscus	It feels as if further force could collapse the joint	Axial compression of the human cervical spine	As with full flexion or extension of the stifle in the presence of a meniscal lesion
Soft tissue apposition	Produced by 2 muscle bulks coming in contact with one another. Motion is stopped by impedance of soft tissues	It feels as if more motion could be obtained of you could apply more force	Stifle flexion	As in the case of obesity-related restrictions to truncall flexion or side flexion
Boggy	Produced by viscous fluid (eg, blood)	It feel as if further force could burst the joint	Never normal	As per description–blood in a joint
Spasm	Produced by a reflexive and reactive muscle contraction in response to irritation of the nociceptors predominantly in articular structures or muscles	It feels as if further force could damage blood vessels	Never normal	As with stifle extension in the case of an acute CCL tear
Empty	Lack of an end feel entirely. No tissue resistance is detected	Nothing. The patient cannot tolerate more ROM dude to pain	Never normal. Usually indicative of a serious pathologic condition	As in the case of an intra-articular fracture, tumor or cyst

Modified from Magee DJ, Zachazewski JE, Quillen WS. Scientific Foundations and Principles of Practice in Musculoskeletal Rehabilitation. Saunders Elsevier, St Louis, 2007.

given to additional tests or factors (such as pain) and noting of changes or differences (ie, from side to side).[30–33] Petersen and Hayes (2000) reported that the presence of pain is more associated with abnormal-pathological end feels than the normal end feels in shoulder and knees of human patients.[34] This finding was also noted in another study that evaluated the cervical spine[35] where combining the assessment of pain provocation and asymmetry of passive intervertebral mobility testing yielded favorable interrater reliability. A biomechanical study also concluded that in elderly patients with unilateral chronic low back pain, muscle tone, and stiffness of paravertebral muscles on the painful side are higher than for those on the nonpainful side.[36] Accurate detection of end feels seems to improve with clinician experience. Kawamura and colleagues,[37] in 2020, utilized an end feel simulator to determine that years of clinical experience and conscious effort to perceive end feels yielded a higher proportion of correct answers compared with less experienced clinicians. Taken as a composite, asymmetry of biomechanical properties, pain, and the evaluation of multiple factors should be noted by clinicians as part of the physical examination in order to adequately interpret end feels and their relevance.

Palpation

In addition to using palpation to determine end feels and stiffness of a joint, palpation to determine muscle symmetry as well as lowered pain threshold is common practice in both human and animal medicine. Palpation is considered to be a key outcome measure and assessment tool for equine rehabilitation professionals.[38] Manual palpation by veterinary physiotherapists has been shown to have excellent interrater reliability when using a categorical scoring system for the determination of mechanical nociception threshold responses for back pain in horses.[39] Back pain in horses can be differentiated by severity of pain response to back palpation, back muscle hypertonicity, and thoracolumbar joint stiffness.[40]

A palpation scale was used in the Merrifield-Jones and colleagues[39] (2019) study that was modified from an earlier scale utilized in a study by Varcoe-Cock and colleagues (2006)[41] (**Table 3**). A similar scale or study that evaluated palpation scoring in dogs could not be found on review of available literature.

Beyond palpation for muscle tone, palpation can also detect pain in other soft tissue structures such as tendons or ligaments. Focal tenderness on palpation of tendons is

Table 3
Manual palpation scale for equine practice

Score	Description
0	Soft, low tone
1	Normal
2	Increased muscle tone but not painful
3	Increased muscle tone and/or painful (slight associated spasm on palpation, no associated movement)
4	Painful (associated spasm on palpation with associated local movement, ie, pelvic tilt, extension response)
5	Very painful (spasm plus behaviour response to palpation, ie, ears flat back, kicking)

With permission from: Merrifield-Jones M, Tabor G, Williams J. Inter- and Intra-Rater Reliability of Soft Tissue Palpation Scoring in the Equine Thoracic Epaxial Region. J Equine Vet Sci. 2019 Dec;83:102812.

a common finding in tendon lesions, and sprained ligaments in both human and veterinary practice.[42-45] Combined with other clinical findings, pain on palpation contributes to the reliability of a physical diagnosis.[46]

SUMMARY

Manual treatment will be determined after a thorough neuromusculoskeletal assessment by a qualified practitioner. This will include using many skills including clinical reasoning, thorough observational assessment, and manual evaluation. When putting all the gathered information together, it should guide the manual therapy treatment plans. The skills discussed in this article are foundational stepping stones for practitioners when determining when, where, how, and which manual therapies to use as treatment techniques in canine rehabilitation.

DISCLOSURE

The authors have no commercial or financial interests to disclose.

DECLARATION OF INTERESTS

None.

CLINICS CARE POINTS

- Manual therapy treatments should not be provided without a skilled evaluation of the animal and its specific tissues.
- Advanced training is required to acquire manual assessment and treatment skills.
- Bayesian clinical reasoning further enables accurate interpretation of assessment finding.

REFERENCES

1. Jones MA, Rivett DA. Introduction to clinical reasoning. In: Jones MA, Rivett DA, editors. Clinical reasoning for manual therapists. Edinburgh: Butterworth Heinemann; 2004. p. 3–24.
2. Bialosky JE, Beneciuk JM, Bishop MD, et al. Unraveling the Mechanisms of Manual Therapy: Modeling an Approach. J Orthop Sports Phys Ther 2018; 48(1):8–18.
3. Jiandani MP, Mhatre BS. Physical therapy diagnosis: how is it different? J Postgrad Med 2018;64(2):69–72.
4. Wikipedia. Bayesian probability. Available at: https://en.wikipedia.org/wiki/Bayesian_probability. Accessed November 18, 2022.
5. Khan S, Freeman P. Bayesian clinical reasoning in the first opinion approach to a dog with suspected thoracolumbar pain. J Small Anim Pract 2022;63(12):853–7.
6. Berman CF, Lobetti RG, Lindquist E. Comparison of clinical findings in 293 dogs with suspect acute pancreatitis: Different clinical presentation with left lobe, right lobe or diffuse involvement of the pancreas. J S Afr Vet Assoc 2020. https://doi.org/10.4102/jsava.v91i0.2022.
7. Higgs J, Jones M. Clinical reasoning in the health professions. In: Higgs J, Jones M, Loftus S, et al, editors. Clinical reasoning in the health professions. Edinburgh: Butterworth Heinemann; 2008. p. 24.

8. Yeung E, Woods N, Dubrowski A, et al. Establishing assessment criteria for clinical reasoning in orthopedic manual physical therapy: a consensus-building study. J Man Manip Ther 2015 Feb;23(1):27–36.

9. Gillette R, Graig T. Canine locomotion analysis. In: Millis D, Levine D, editors. Canine rehabilitation and physical therapy. Amsterdam: Elsevier; 2014. p. 201–10.

10. Mondino A, Wagner G, Russell K, et al. Static posturography as a novel measure of the effects of aging on postural control in dogs. PLoS One 2022;17(7): e0268390.

11. Lasceles BD, Roe SC, Smith E, et al. Evaluation of a pressure walkway system for measurement of vertical limb forces in clinically normal dogs. Am J Vet Res 2006; 67:277–82.

12. DeCamp CE. Kinetic and kinematic gait analysis and the assessment of lameness in the dog. Vet Clin North Am Small Anim Pract 1997;27(4):825–40.

13. Budsberg SC, Verstaete MC, Brown J, et al. Vertical loading rates in clinically normal dogs at a trot. Am J Vet Res 1995;56:1275–80.

14. Gillette RL, Angle TC. Recent developments in canine locomotor analysis: a review. Vet J 2008;178:165–76.

15. Mölsä SH, Hyytiäinen HK, Hielm-Björkman AK, et al. Long-term functional outcome after surgical repair of cranial cruciate ligament disease in dogs. BMC Vet Res 2014;10:266.

16. Evans R, Horstman C, Conzemius M. Accuracy and optimization of force platform gait analysis in Labradors with cranial cruciate disease evaluated at a walking gait. Vet Surg 2005;34(5):445–9.

17. Poy NSJ, DeCamp CE, Bennett RL, et al. Additional kinematic variables to describe differences in the trot between clinically normal dogs and dogs with hip dysplasia. Am J Vet Res 2000;61(8):974–8.

18. Bockstahler BA, Vobornik A, Müller M, et al. Compensatory load redistribution in naturally occurring osteoarthritis of the elbow joint and induced weight-bearing lameness of the forelimbs compared with clinically sound dogs. Vet J 2009; 180:202–12.

19. Moses PA, McGowan CM. Neurological and muscular conditions. In: McGowan CM, Goff L, Stubbs N, editors. Animal physiotherapy: assessment, treatment and rehabilitation of animals. Ames, Iowa: Blackwell Publishing; 2007. p. p.115–117.

20. Amaral Marrero NP, Thomovsky SA, Linder JE, et al. Static body weight distribution and girth measurements over time in dogs after acute thoracolumbar intervertebral disc extrusion. Front Vet Sci 2022;9:877402.

21. Cyriax J. Textbook of orthopaedic medicine volume I. Diagnosis of soft tissue lesions. 8th ed. London: Bailliere Tindall; 1982.

22. Cyriax JH, Cyriax PJ. Illustrated manual of orthopaedic medicine. 2nd ed. Oxford, UK: Butterworth Heinemann; 1993.

23. Magee DJ. Orthopedic physical assessment. 5th ed. St. Louis, MO: Saunders Elsevier; 2008. p. 1–70.

24. Pellecchia GL, Paolino J, Connell J. Intertester reliability of the Cyriax evaluation in assessing patients with shoulder pain. J Orthop Sports Phys Ther 1996; 23(1):34–8.

25. Hanchard NC, Howe TE, Gilbert MM. Diagnosis of shoulder pain by history and selective tissue tension: agreement between assessors. J Orthop Sports Phys Ther 2005;35(3):147–53.

26. Storheil B, Klouman E, Holmvik S, et al. Intertester reliability of shoulder complaints diagnoses in primary health care. Scand J Prim Health Care 2016;34(3): 224–31.
27. Jaegger G, Marcellin-Little DJ, Levine D. Reliability of goniometry in labrador retrievers. Am J Vet Res 2002;63(7):979–86.
28. Thomas TM, Marcellin-Little DJ, Roe SC, et al. Comparison of measurements obtained by use of an electrogoniometer and a universal plastic goniometer for the assessment of joint motion in dogs Todd. Am J Vet Res 2006;67:1974–9.
29. Magee DJ, Zachazewski JE, Quillen WS. Scientific Foundations and Principles of practice in musculoskeletal rehabilitation. St. Louis: Saunders Elsevier; 2007. p. 518–9.
30. Chesworth BM, MacDermid JC, Roth JH, et al. Movement diagram and "end-feel" reliability when measuring passive lateral rotation of the shoulder in patients with shoulder pathology. Phys Ther 1998;78(6):593–601.
31. Hayes KW, Petersen CM. Reliability of assessing end-feel and pain and resistance sequence in subjects with painful shoulders and knees. J Orthop Sports Phys Ther 2001;31(8):432–45.
32. Manning DM, Dedrick GS, Sizer PS, et al. Reliability of a seated three-dimensional passive intervertebral motion test for mobility, end-feel, and pain provocation in patients with cervicalgia. J Man Manip Ther 2012;20(3):135–41.
33. Jonsson A, Rasmussen-Barr E. Intra- and inter-rater reliability of movement and palpation tests in patients with neck pain: a systematic review. Physiother Theory Pract 2018;34(3):165–80.
34. Petersen CM, Hayes KW. Construct validity of Cyriax's selective tension examination: association of end-feels with pain at the knee and shoulder. J Orthop Sports Phys Ther 2000;30(9):512–21 [discussion: 522–527].
35. Hariharan KV, Timko MG, Bise CG, et al. Inter-examiner reliability study of physical examination procedures to assess the cervical spine. Chiropr Man Therap 2021;29(1):20.
36. Wu Z, Ye X, Ye Z, et al. Asymmetric biomechanical properties of the paravertebral muscle in elderly patients with unilateral chronic low back pain: a preliminary study. Front Bioeng Biotechnol 2022;10:814099.
37. Kawamura H, Tasaka S, Ikeda A, et al. Ability to categorize end-feel joint movement according to years of clinical experience: an experiment with an end-feel simulator. J Phys Ther Sci 2020;32(4):297–302.
38. Tabor G, Nankervis K, Fernandes J, et al. Generation of domains for the equine musculoskeletal rehabilitation outcome score: development by expert consensus. Animals (Basel) 2020;10(2):203.
39. Merrifield-Jones M, Tabor G, Williams J. Inter- and intra-rater reliability of soft tissue palpation scoring in the equine thoracic epaxial region. J Equine Vet Sci 2019;83:102812.
40. Mayaki AM, Abdul Razak IS, Adzahan NM, et al. Clinical assessment and grading of back pain in horses. J Vet Sci 2020;21(6):e82.
41. Varcoe-Cocks K, Sagar KN, Jeffcott LB, et al. Pressure algometry to quantify muscle pain in racehorses with suspected sacroiliac dysfunction. Equine Vet J 2006;38(6):558–62.
42. Hamilton B, Purdam C. Patellar tendinosis as an adaptive process: a new hypothesis. Br J Sports Med 2004;38(6):758–61.
43. Carvalho CD, Cohen C, Belangero PS, et al. Supraspinatus muscle tendon lesion and its relationship with long head of the biceps lesion. Rev Bras Ortop (Sao Paulo) 2020;55(3):329–38.

44. Netterström-Wedin F, Bleakley C. Diagnostic accuracy of clinical tests assessing ligamentous injury of the ankle syndesmosis: a systematic review with meta-analysis. Phys Ther Sport 2021;49:214–26.
45. von Pfeil DJF, Steinberg EJ, Dycus D. Arthroscopic tenotomy for treatment of biceps tendon luxation in two apprehension police dogs. J Am Vet Med Assoc 2020;257(11):1157–64.
46. Rosas S, Krill MK, Amoo-Achampong K, et al. A practical, evidence-based, comprehensive (PEC) physical examination for diagnosing pathology of the long head of the biceps. J Shoulder Elbow Surg 2017;26(8):1484–92.

Veterinary Spinal Manipulative Therapy or Animal Chiropractic in Veterinary Rehabilitation

Rosemary J. LoGiudice, DVM, DACVSMR, CCRT, CVA, CVSMT, FCoAC[a,b,]*,
Pedro Luis Rivera, DVM, FACFN, DACVSMR, FCoAC[b,c]

KEYWORDS

- Animal chiropractic • Spinal manipulative therapy • Veterinary rehabilitation
- Complementary and alternative and integrative therapies • Neuromuscular plasticity
- Kinesiopathology • Hypomobility • Vertebral subluxation complex

KEY POINTS

- Veterinary spinal manipulative therapy (SMT), or animal chiropractic (AC), is a valuable receptor-based health care modality, that can be incorporated into veterinary rehabilitation protocols as a diagnostic tool as well as a treatment modality, especially for patients with lower back pain, as chiropractic is being used in human healthcare.
- Identifying any kinesiopathology or hypomobility of a patient is an essential aspect of AC.
- Appropriately trained clinicians can safely, efficiently, and competently assess a patient's presentation and provide appropriate treatment that may improve outcomes, based on sound neuroanatomical and biomechanical changes.
- When performed by appropriately trained and licensed practitioners; AC has a lower incidence of injury or adverse reactions than many standard therapies and medications.
- A practitioner must thoroughly assess the patient to know if AC is an appropriate therapy and must understand the functional changes that an adjustment may have.

 Video content accompanies this article at http://www.vetsmall.theclinics.com.

INTRODUCTION

Veterinary rehabilitation is a multimodal diagnostic and treatment approach that is routinely recommended and provided to patients. One therapeutic modality that may be beneficial (diagnostically and therapeutically) is veterinary spinal

[a] Animal Rehabilitation Therapy & Sports Medicine, Yorkville, IL, USA; [b] Healing Oasis Wellness Center, Sturtevant, WI, USA; [c] Healing Oasis Veterinary Hospital, 2555 Wisconsin Street, Sturtevant, WI 53177-8100, USA
* Corresponding author. 2555 Wisconsin Street, Sturtevant, WI 53177-8100.
E-mail address: animalrehabtherapy@gmail.com

manipulative therapy (VSMT) or animal chiropractic (AC). AC is a receptor-based health-care modality being provided more frequently in veterinary practices. The goal of rehabilitation as described by the American Association of Rehabilitation Veterinarians is to achieve the highest level of function, independence, and quality of life possible for the patient. This article will explore using AC as a valuable modality in veterinary rehabilitation.

Although some veterinary schools provide basic information on several integrative health-care modalities, none offers in-depth postgraduate education. Licensed professionals must seek and complete postgraduate training to understand this health-care modality. All clinicians should strive to understand the mode of action, indications, contraindications, how it affects the patient from the neuro-anatomical and biomechanical point of view, and most importantly, when not to provide the requested modality, as further diagnostics may be indicated.

BRIEF HISTORY

For many centuries, the mobilization of soft tissues and joints has been provided to patients. Still, it was not until the latter part of the 1800s that Dr Daniel D. Palmer developed the term *chiropractic*, and he is considered the father of the chiropractic profession. Chiropractic is a Greek word derived from *cheir*, meaning hand, and *praktike* or *prakticos*, meaning to practice.[1,2] As with any health care modality, the origins are rudimentary and develop from a basic description. During the mid-to-late 1800s, Dr Daniel D. Palmer developed the definition of *chiropractic vertebral subluxation (CVS)*, to be defined as *a partial separation of two articular surfaces*.[3,4] Unfortunately, the description of *bone out of place*[5] may have been incorrectly attributed to Dr Palmer.[3] The simplistic theory of CVS should not be surprising, because during the same period, human medical treatments and services ranged from toxic purgatives and herbal concoctions, magnetic therapy, to bloodletting, as some examples. The National Institutes of Health states that *Chiropractic Science is concerned with investigating the relationship between structure, primarily the spine, and function, primarily the nervous system of the human body in order to restore and preserve its health*.[6] Other definitions can be found in the literature.[3,7–10]

In an article published in JAMA (Journal of the American Medical Association) in 2021, spinal manipulation is a recommended option for patients to seek as an initial treatment of low back pain.[11] Sharon Willoughby, DVM, DC, who trained under Thomas Offen, DC, is credited with starting the first AC training of modern days in the United States.[12,13]

Spinal manipulative therapy (SMT), chiropractic, or AC differs from other manual therapies in that it provides and utilizes adjustments. An adjustment is a high-velocity low amplitude (HVLA) thrust into a specific osseous segmental contact in a specific line of drive (LOD) to the motion unit.[4,14,15] A motion unit comprises 2 adjacent bones, which includes the intra-articular and periarticular components of the joint.[4,8,16] The LOD is specific to the joint plane as all motion units have their particular anatomic range of motion.[4,14,15] AC can be applied to any synovial joint, not just those from the spine (**Fig. 1**A, B).

The early simplistic explanation of how the adjustment *worked was based on restoring the biomechanics of the vertebral column and indirectly influences neurologic functions*.[2] Even though the cited author used the term indirectly, an adjustment affects the nervous system and its operations directly and indirectly.[4]

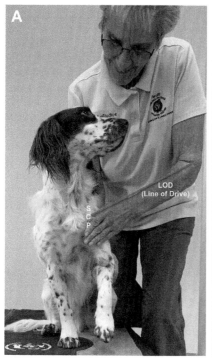
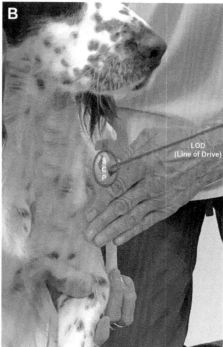

Fig. 1. (*A*) Setup for evaluating and adjusting an external rotation restriction (hypomobility) of the left humeral head (glenohumeral joint). (*B*) Close-up of the setup for external rotation restriction (hypomobility) of the left humeral head-demonstrating segmental contact point (greater tubercle) and contact point (guarded thumb as well) as LOD.

What Is Included in an Animal Chiropractic Evaluation?

A proper AC evaluation should include the following:

- Thorough history
- Understanding the type of training or competitive activities in which the patient is currently or has engaged
- Review of previous records or diagnostics (not just reading the reports)
- Gait evaluation
- Complete physical examination, including a thorough neurologic and musculoskeletal system evaluation
- Motion palpation of the entire patient, not just the affected area
- Providing and explaining the valid differential diagnosis to the client before delivering the adjustment. Please note that depending on the differential diagnoses, further diagnostics might be indicated *before* providing an adjustment
- Treat the patient (provide adjustment[s]) *if indicated*
- Describe to the owner the changes that may occur after the adjustment
- Provide a recheck time and what to do at home, such as take-home exercises as an example
- Maintain complete medical records (SOAP [Subjective, Objective, Assessment, Progress Plan] format)

What Does Animal Chiropractic Assess?

AC assesses for hypomobility in a specific motion unit. An old term, which some professionals are still using to describe a hypomobile unit, is *subluxation*.[2,15,17] The term *subluxation* describes a vertebral joint dysfunction used to *designate contiguous vertebrae that displayed an abnormal positional relationship* and *is a complex of functional and/or structural and/or pathological articular changes that compromise neural integrity and may influence organ system function and general health*.[2,15,17] Another description that academia and researchers have developed is *vertebral subluxation complex* (VSC).[18,19] VSC describes the changes of global and dynamic changes of hypomobility among many tissues, including but not limited to the neuromusculoskeletal systems. However, VSC still uses the term *subluxation*, which brings confusion.[18,20] A fascinating aspect of the VSC cascade is the identification of kinesiopathology as the main common denominator for this complex. The authors recommend using the term of *hypomobility* rather than *subluxation* to avoid confusion and miscommunications (**Fig. 2**).

How Do We Find a Hypomobile Motion Unit?

Motion units with an aberrant range of motion (ROM) can be identified by assessing for heat, tenderness, and hypomobility.[16] The clinician assesses for heat and tenderness by utilizing their hands to statically evaluate the hypomobile region.[16,21] In addition, they may verify the heat changes by appropriate use of thermography.[22] The last and most important method to assess for hypomobility is motion palpation of the affected area. Motion palpation helps the clinician compare the movement or restriction of the joint when comparing the cranial to caudal aspects or side-to-side differences; in essence, comparing its global motion.[23–26] To correctly assess the specific joint motion, the clinician must be very well versed in the basic osseous anatomy, surrounding muscles, and their primary innervation.

As part of the examination, the patient's gait can provide visual information of their normal active range of motion.[27] After that, the clinician needs to assess for passive ROM (PROM) to the joint's end feel or endplay (end of PROM) of the motion unit (**Fig. 3**). It is not our goal to review how joints move within a 3-dimensional complex but to describe the basic joint global movement briefly.

Joint motion is evaluated within the above-described ROMs, reaching the end of PROM or *endplay*. Once at the *end-play*, the adjustment (HVLA) is provided, which would bring this joint into an area of movement described as the paraphysiological space.[28,29] If the clinician uses excessive force or amplitude when providing the adjustment, the possibility of injuring the patient increases exponentially.

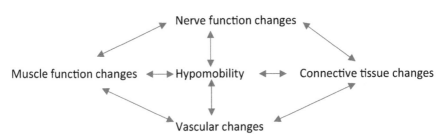

Fig. 2. Flow chart showing changes that can lead to hypomobility. Chemical, physiological, developmental, and inflammatory changes are not included.

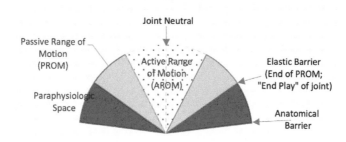

Fig. 3. AC joint motion.

It is crucial for the clinician to rule out functional or pathologic changes that may affect any intra-articular or periarticular components. These components include but are not limited to aberrant developmental anatomy of the joint, adhesions within the synovial folds, joint capsule, and surrounding muscles, tendons, and ligaments. As clinicians, an appropriate differential diagnosis with a thoughtful diagnostic workup should be included. Motion palpation is crucial to identify joint restrictions and commensurable with the clinician's training and experience.[30–35]

Importance of Addressing Changes to Hypomobile Motion Units

A restricted motion unit can start a vicious cycle by decreasing afferent input to the central nervous system (CNS), not to mention the degenerative changes that occur from lack of movement.[36–38] It is essential to remember that afferent stimulation from any receptor affects the local area, spinal cord region, and suprasegmental areas of the nervous system.[33,39–41] Other changes secondary to hypomobility involving blood pressure and nociceptive modulation have been published.[42,43]

It is crucial to understand that joint hypomobility may have a cascade effect influencing local receptors (Golgi tendon organs, muscle spindle cells, nociceptors, and joint mechanoreceptors as examples), as well as the muscles, tendons, and ligaments surrounding the joint.[44,45] Depending on the motion unit affected, vertebral versus extremities, focus should be on the components and boundaries of the said motion unit. The components of the Intervertebral Foramen (IVF) are something to be aware of when addressing hypomobilities of articular facets (**Box 1**). Secondary changes such as decrease ROM as well as decreased performance are some of the clinical presentations from hypomobilities. Clinicians must keep in mind several cascades or responses, such as somato-visceral, somato-autonomic, and viscero-somatic, to name a few, to help them prepare a valid differential diagnosis. It is suggested that the reader review these topics in appropriate veterinary and chiropractic texts addressing pertinent neuroanatomy.

What Happens When an Adjustment Is Provided?

The goal of AC is to bring motion into a joint that has not been moving correctly through its normal ROM if indicated. As discussed in the previous section, hypomobility leads to degenerative changes. A proper adjustment causes the following changes:[8,36,45–48]

- Gapping of the specific joint.[36,45,49,50]
- Breaks up adhesions that have developed due to hypomobility.[36,47,50]

Box 1
Components of the intervertebral foramen[2,98,99]

Dorsal root ganglia

Spinal nerve with its peripheral branches

Dural sleeve

Cerebrospinal fluid

Vascular components

Lymphatics

Connective tissues (including fat)

Transforaminal or intervertebral foraminal ligaments

- The above changes help to release entrapment or extrapment of the synovial folds.[50–52]
- Stimulation peripheral receptors.[50,53,54]
- Stimulation of the afferent fibers, and their postsynaptic connections.[48,53,55]
- Stimulation of the spinal cord, with their divergent connections.[48,50,53,55]
- Stimulation of the cortex or upper motor neurons, and as such, improving modulatory efferent responses.[48]
- Proper neuronal stimulation, which is crucial for developing appropriate plasticity, and the ability to decrease stress levels.[56,57]

Secondary changes to an adjustment as listed above include but are not limited to improvement of somatosensory cortical stimulation, improvement on nociceptive (pain) control, muscle strength, neuromuscular modulation, and neuronal plasticity, as examples. Neuronal plasticity is the ability of the cell to adapt or mold to their presynaptic stimulation. Neuronal plasticity allows for stronger and long-lasting connections[58,59] (see **Fig. 3**).

Efficacy and Safety

There have been several articles published showing the efficacy of AC.[22,54,55,60] Most articles published discussing effectiveness and safety have been from human research, reporting a very low incidence of injuries when provided by licensed and trained professionals.[61–65] Unfortunately, some authors still misuse, misinterpret, or confuse terms when citing articles, which should encourage the reader to read the entire article, not just the abstract.[66] Some articles have been published describing erroneous information, such as what lay people or other nonchiropractic professionals are doing being described as chiropractic adjustments.[67,68] This latter unethical behavior, disrespect to other professions, and outright misinformation should be considered fraudulent.[69] Other national agencies have published information showing the statistical significance of SMT over other treatment therapies[70,71] (**Figs. 4 and 5**).

Indications

AC treatments are sought by clients because of the positive results that their owners have had with their chiropractors addressing unresolved, or sometimes obscure, lameness or unexplained discomfort or pain plaguing them. The clients recognize that if it works for them, it should work for their loved pets. From the rehabilitation point of view, AC may help to improve the strength, stability, and motion of specific joints by

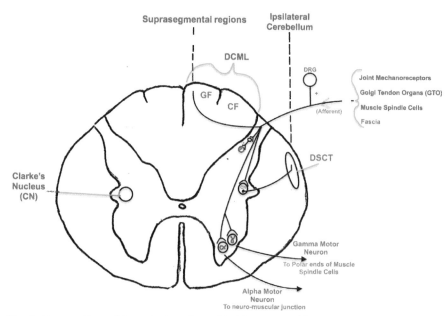

Fig. 4. Cross section of the spinal cord provided by Dr. Arnaldo Monge. Divergent connections added by authors. -, inhibitory interneuron; +, afferent excitatory large diameter fiber; CF, cuneate fasciculus; DRG, dorsal root ganglia; DSCT, dorsal spinocerebellar tract; GF, gracile fasciculus; Red P, second order neuron of spinothalamic tract being inhibited by an interneuron.

addressing hypomobilities and identifying the longitudinal level of the lesion (LLL; see **Fig. 3**).

Contraindications

A common-sense approach to treatment is highly recommended, with complete diagnostics when indicated. A complete evaluation should be provided, as discussed in a previous section titled, *What is included in an AC evaluation*. Some contraindications may include but are not limited to organ failure, neoplasia, fever, hemorrhage, fracture, acute disc protrusion or extrusion, and immune-mediated problems.

Using Animal Chiropractic in Veterinary Rehabilitation

Veterinary rehabilitation patients include a broad selection of animals, including preoperative and postoperative surgical patients, neurologic, and musculoskeletal cases. In addition, normal, geriatric/senior, athletes, or service animals may also benefit from rehabilitation. We suggest that virtually every dog is an athlete. For example, consider the athleticism required for a small dog who is a companion to jump onto a couch several times higher than the dog's height to sit next to its owner. Because older animals are often presented for rehabilitation, we should understand the difference between the terms *geriatric* and *senior*. There has been considerable information published about canine aging.[72–74] It is not uncommon for veterinarians to classify dogs as senior at a younger age than do clients.[75]

As was previously described, a thorough physical examination, complete neurologic evaluation, and motion palpation to assess joint mobility precede any AC treatment. The authors maintain that one value for incorporating AC into every

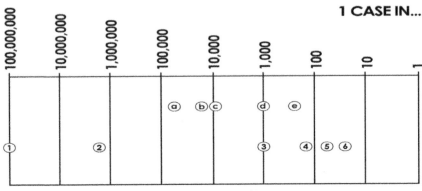

Fig. 5. The items discussed above demonstrate the low risk of spinal manipulation compared to surgical and medical treatments, as well as occurrences. Graph created by Dr. Gregory Cramer (Dean of Research at National Univ. of Health Sciences, Lombard, IL) with information gathered from the Bandolier Website (https://ebm.bmj.com/), an evidence-based newsletter, and other published articles. (Reprinted with permission. Citation: Cramer, G; 2017 The clinical anatomy of spinal manipulation. Study Guide for Veterinary SMT Program, The Healing Oasis, Sturtevant, Wisconsin; 16pp.)

rehabilitation evaluation is that hypomobility can be detected and addressed at the functional level before pathologic changes with its clinical signs develop. The ultimate goal is to maintain the patient's optimal functional neurologic and musculoskeletal systems to improve their conditioning and performance. Still, any hypomobilities found should be mentioned and discussed, allowing the clients to decide if they want their dog treated. Not every client understands the potential value of appropriate AC adjustments, so this opportunity to educate the client should not be missed.

AC can also be used as part of our diagnostic evaluations. When asked to examine a patient for a specific issue, the entire animal, not just the area in question, should be evaluated. When considering an affected area, the AC clinicians should consider the innervation of both agonistic and antagonistic muscles related to the hypomobility. As with any lameness or biomechanical condition, the LLL that may be responsible for the presenting clinical issue should be determined. Suppose we focus only on the presenting clinical issue and work to improve that with our rehabilitation therapies but do not find and address the LLL. In that case, the clinical problem may temporarily improve but return when the animal resumes regular activity.

Next, some examples of common issues that may be improved by incorporating AC into veterinary rehabilitation will be discussed.

Incontinence (Urinary and/or Fecal)

Incontinence is an issue that plagues many dogs, especially as they age, and is considered to be a primary reason for the euthanizing of geriatric dogs.[76] The nerves responsible for both sensory and motor functions of micturition originate from the lower lumbar and sacral spinal segments. Sensory pathways of micturition and defecation are primarily through the pelvic and pudendal nerves, originating from the spinal cord segments S1-S3, and the hypogastric nerve, originating from segments L1-L4. The sympathetic motor function of micturition to the bladder includes the splanchnic nerves, originating from segments L1-L4, with the hypogastric nerve. The external urethral sphincter innervation is primarily through the pudendal nerve.[77] Control of defecation also relies on sensory and motoric neurologic activity, including the pelvic and the hypogastric nerves.[78] Hypomobilities of the lumbar spine have been correlated to urinary incontinence in dogs.[79] In addition to sensory and motor control, a dog must posture comfortably to urinate and defecate properly. Caudal lumbo-sacro-pelvic orthopedic restriction, including osteoarthritis and pain, may prevent the dog from correct posturing and may thereby contribute significantly to incontinence.[16,80] If the hypomobilities causing pain are addressed, then the neurologic function and improvement of incontinence can be achieved.[79,81]

Lumbar/Sacroiliac or Low Back Pain

As discussed in the previous section, caudal lumbar pain may prevent the dog from posturing correctly to urinate or defecate. Our goal is to describe ways in which AC can help improve lumbar and/or sacroiliac pain, thereby improving mobility and function of the region. *The sacroiliac joint (SIJ) is often overlooked as a source of chronic low back pain. The SIJ is a diarthrodial synovial joint that is thought to have a role in ambulation.*[82]

Veterinary rehabilitation practitioners trained in AC must emphasize the correlation between motion and its effects on neuromuscular plasticity.[83] When a clinical presentation points to lower back discomfort, the lumbar, lumbosacral, and sacroiliac areas may be of particular concern. In the past, evaluating and trying to maintain optimal sacroiliac and lumbosacral joint mobility has been based primarily on anecdotal and clinical experience and extrapolating from human and equine findings.[1,11] If we further extrapolate from research done with horses, AC is an effective therapeutic modality to improve the mechanical nociceptive thresholds in healthy animals exhibiting no clinical signs of low back (lumbar) pain.[84] Although it is clinically accepted that SIJ disease contributes to lower back/lumbosacral area pain in dogs, retrospective research published in June 2022 correlates the computed tomographic (CT), and MRI characteristics that are found in humans with SIJ disease are also common in large breed dogs.[85]

SMT is recommended by the American College of Physicians and the American Medical Association to treat people with acute or subacute low back pain.[11,86] Thorough knowledge of the anatomy of the articulations involved in the lumbar, lumbosacral, and SIJs as well as of the neurology in the area is necessary to properly access and correlate the physical findings when performing motion palpation and before performing any adjustments. In addition to lumbosacral and sacroiliac pain and hypomobility, consider AC for dogs with back pain and those with intervertebral disc disease that may not be appropriate surgical candidates[87] (**Fig. 6A–C**).

Pelvic Limb Lameness

Cranial cruciate ligament disease is a common presentation of pelvic limb lameness in dogs.[88,89] Rehabilitation therapy is often sought as an element of the treatment of cranial cruciate ligament disease, either before or after surgery or as conservative management.[90] One of the things the authors encourage our clients to do is *prehabilitation*, which is important to help improve strength, stability, and conditioning of the patient before surgery, and may also result in improved postoperative recovery. As

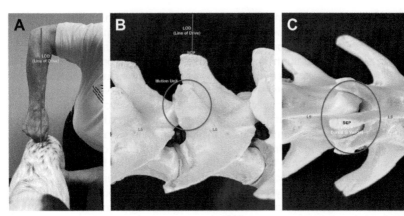

Fig. 6. (*A*) Demonstration of the setup to perform caudal lumbar spine motion palpation and subsequent adjustment, if necessary. (*B*) Lateral view of the osseous anatomy of the L6 dorsal to ventral motion palpation and hypomobility adjustment setup; showing the LOD, segmental contact point (SCP) (dorsal spinous process), and the motion unit (L^ on L5 articular facets). (*C*) Dorsal-ventral view of the osseous anatomy of the L6 dorsal to ventral motion palpation and hypomobility adjustment setup; showing the LOD, SCP (dorsal spinous process), and the motion unit (L6 on L5 articular facets).

veterinarians, we should understand the importance of treating an injured area in question and determine what may have initiated the cause, potential causes, or contributing factors that resulted in the clinical injury.

Consideration on maintaining optimal strength, flexibility, and function of the muscles responsible for proper stifle joint mobility and stability is a must. However, please remember that muscles cannot function properly without healthy and appropriate neurologic information. The nerves innervating the muscles responsible for pelvic limb function originate from the lumbosacral plexus. If we consider the stifle joint, from the anatomic standpoint, most of the extensor muscles (quadriceps muscle group, cranial head of the sartorius) are innervated by the femoral nerve, originating from the spinal nerves L4-6. The tensor fasciae latae, which also acts as a stifle joint extensor, is innervated by the cranial gluteal nerve, which originates from L6-S1. Some of the stifle joint flexor muscles (biceps femoris, semitendinosus, semimembranosus) are innervated by the sciatic nerve, which originates from the last 2 lumbar and first 2 sacral spinal nerves. In contrast, the caudal head of the sartorius muscle, which assists in the flexion of the stifle joint, is innervated by the femoral nerve (saphenous branch), which originates from the L4-6 spinal nerves.[89,91] From this information, we should be able to deduce that maintaining optimal vertebral mobility should assist in providing maximal neuromuscular plasticity and function. We have described local neuromuscular effects here and do not include the effects that maintaining optimal vertebral mobility may have on the ideal function of the spinal tracts (see **Fig. 3**).

Thoracic Limb Lameness

Determining the source of forelimb lameness can be challenging. It is crucial to determine the LLL, which may be the underlying cause of the clinical symptom(s). Most of the muscles responsible for the function of the thoracic limb are innervated by branches from the brachial plexus (originating from the secondary curvature) with the spinal nerve levels of C(5)6-T1(2). Other important nerves affecting the thoracic limb include the spinal accessory (brachiocephalicus, omotransversarius, and trapezius muscles as examples), the long thoracic (C7) (serratus ventralis m.), and the thoracodorsal (C8-T1 latissimus dorsi m.).[91]

Another diagnosis that may present as thoracic limb lameness includes *nerve root syndrome* or *root signature*. Some of the causes to consider regarding nerve root syndrome in dogs include foraminal stenosis, disc herniation, nerve entrapment, and nerve sheath tumors. There are several biomechanical and biochemical factors that result from the compression or irritation of the affected cervical nerve root. Still, all the changes appear due to changes in the microcirculation of the affected nerve.[92] If the restriction of the involved intervertebral foramina can be improved, allowing improved circulation of the component going through the IVF, then improvement of the symptoms may be expected. This was the case with one of the authors' dogs, who would present with occasional, significant left thoracic limb lameness with minimal weight-bearing, negative to pain during limb palpation, and no radiographic findings, which would resolve within minutes of adjusting the C5-C6 motion unit (**Fig. 7**A–D, Video 1).

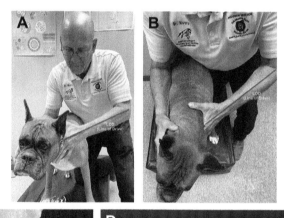

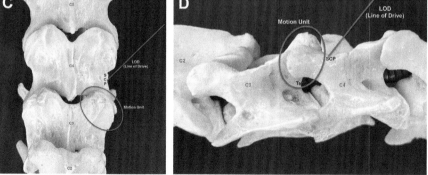

Fig. 7. (*A*) Demonstration of the setup to perform cervical spine motion palpation and subsequent adjustment, if necessary. (*B*) Demonstration of the setup to perform cervical spine motion palpation and subsequent adjustment, if necessary.(*C*) Dorsal-ventral view of the osseous anatomy of the C4 motion palpation and hypomobility adjustment setup; showing LOD SCP (lamina pedicle junction), and the motion unit (C4 on C3). (*D*) Lateral view of the cervical osseous anatomy showing the SCP (lamina pedicle junction), LOD, and the motion unit (C4 on C3).

Box 2
Resources

American Association of Rehabilitation Veterinarians: www.rehabvets.org

American College of Veterinary Sports Medicine and Rehabilitation: www.vsmr.org

American Holistic Veterinary Medical Association (An AVMA-House of Delegates recognized organization): www.ahvma.org

American Veterinary Chiropractic Association: www.animalchiropractic.org

College of Animal Chiropractors: www.collegeofanimalchiropractors.org

International Veterinary Chiropractic Association: https://ivca.de/

Please note that the above-listed resources are membership organizations, not policing, licensing, or accrediting agencies.

Fascia

Another critical aspect of veterinary rehabilitation to be considered is how AC can influence the fascial system and how it can affect mobility. Fascia is a strong connective tissue structure that is richly innervated and serves as a source of afferent information from different types of receptors (encapsulated and nonencapsulated) that enhances proprioception at the central level.[93,94] Fascia also connects muscles and visceral organs in an orderly fashion.[52] Because of this extensive organization and the vast number of receptors, fascia plays an important role in maintaining coordinated gaits, mobility, and the overall function of the musculoskeletal system.[94–96]

SUMMARY

Properly applied AC can be safe and effective.[61,62,97] Only licensed health-care professionals who have successfully completed extensive postgraduate training should offer AC.

As we initially described, the goal of rehabilitation is to achieve the highest level of function, independence, and quality of life possible for the patient. In this article, we have described that using AC is a valuable modality that by improving afferent input and positive modulation of the ventral horn cells, and their motor neurons, patient strength, stability, and mobility can be positively affected. Patient outcomes, therefore, including improved conditioning, performance, and postoperative recoveries can be enhanced through the inclusion of AC in rehabilitation protocols (**Box 2** - Resources).

CLINICS CARE POINTS

- Always strive to understand the neurologic consequences of an adjustment before addressing the hypomobility.
- Incorporate AC motion palpation whenever possible as part of your full examination of each patient and always motion palpate the entire animal, not just the area of concern.
- Always try to determine the "LLL," the actual inciting cause of the clinical symptom(s), rather than just treating the symptoms.
- Identification of any kinesiopathology or hypomobility of a patient is an essential aspect of AC.
- Never adjust a hypermobile motion unit.

- Some contraindications to AC may include but are not limited to organ failure, neoplasia, fever, hemorrhage, fracture, acute disc protrusion or extrusion, and immune-mediated problems.

DISCLOSURE

No disclosures other than Dr P.L. Rivera is the Program Director and Co-Owner of The Healing Oasis Wellness Center Accredited School and Dr R.J. LoGiudice is a Senior Faculty at the Healing Oasis Wellness Center. No other sponsorships or financial disclosures.

SUPPLEMENTARY DATA

Supplementary data related to this article can be found online at https://doi.org/10.1016/j.cvsm.2023.02.008.

REFERENCES

1. Haussler K. Chiropractic evaluation and management. In: Haussler K, editor. Veterinary clinics of north America equine pracitce: back problems. Philadelphia: Saunders; 1999. p. 197.
2. Willoughby S. Chiropractic care. In: Schoen A, Wynn SG, editors. Complementary and alternative veterinary medicine - principles and practice. St. Louis, Missouri, USA: Mosby; 1998. p. 185–200.
3. Senzon SA. The chiropractic vertebral subluxation part 2: the earliest subluxation theories from 1902 to 1907. J Chiropr Humanit 2018;25:22–35.
4. Gatterman M. What's in a word?. In: Gatterman MI, editor. Foundations of chiropractic - subluxation. 2nd edition. St. Louis, MO, USA: Elsevier/Mosby; 2005. p. 6–18.
5. Boop S, Wheless J, Van Poppel K, et al. Cerebellar seizures. J Neurosurg Pediatr 2013;12:288–92.
6. Brennan B, Rosner A, Demmerle A, et al. Manual healing methods. In: Board NR, editor. Alternative medicine - expanding medical horizons. Chantilly, VA, USA: NIH; 1992. p. 113–57.
7. Available at: https://www.nccih.nih.gov/health/chiropractic-in-depth. Accessed March 14, 2023.
8. Rivera P. Spinal manipulation or animal chiropractic and the musculoskeletal system - its influence in quadruped locomotion. Integrative Veterinary Care Winter 2015;16:52–6.
9. Cleveland A, Phillips R, Clum G. The chiropractic paradigm. In: *Fundamentals of chiropractic*. St. Louis, MO: Mosby; 2003. p. 15–27.
10. Hart J. Analysis and adjustment of vertebral subluxation as a separate and distinct identity for the chiropractic profession: a commentary. J Chiropr Humanit 2016;23:46–52.
11. Traeger AC, Qaseem A, McAuley JH. Low back pain. JAMA 2021;326:286.
12. Animals of. animal chiropractic history. Available at: https://optionsforanimals.com/about-us/history/. Accessed September 11, 2022.
13. UP Organization. The latest news. 2018; Obituary. Available at: https://www.uspolo.org/news-social/news/dr-thomas-offen. Accessed September 11, 2022.

14. Wood TG, Colloca CJ, Matthews R. A pilot randomized clinical trial on the relative effect of instrumental (MFMA) versus manual (HVLA) manipulation in the treatment of cervical spine dysfunction. J Manip Physiol Ther 2001;24:260–71.

15. Leach R. In: The chiropractic theories - a textbook of scientific research. 4th edition. Baltimore, MD: Lippincott Williams & Wilkins; 2004. p. 29–42.

16. Rivera P, LoGiudice R. Veterinary spinal manipulation (animal chiropractic): a functional neuro-anatomical approach to help aging pets requiring palliative or hospice care. JAHVMA 2019;56:41–8.

17. Leach R. General Introduction. In: Leach R, editor. Chiropractic theories - a textbook of scientific research. Baltimore, MD, USA: Lippincott Williams & Wilkins; 2004. p. 3–12.

18. Seaman DRFL. The Vertebral subluxation complex. In: Gatterman M, editor. Foundations of chiropractic - subluxation. 2nd edition. St. Louis, MO, USA: Mosby; 2005. p. 196–226.

19. Cleveland CI. Vertebral subluxation. In: Fundamentals of chiropractic. St. Louis, MO: Mosby; 2003. p. 129–53.

20. Lantz C. The vertebral subluxation complex. Foundations of chiropractic subluxation. St. Louis, MO, USA: Mosby; 1995. p. 150–74.

21. Beynon AM, Hebert JJ, Walker BF. The interrater reliability of static palpation of the thoracic spine for eliciting tenderness and stiffness to test for a manipulable lesion. Chiropr Man Ther 2018;26:49.

22. McQueen EKUS, McQueen MT. Equine performance and autonomic nervous system improvement after joint manipulation: a case study. J Equine Vet Sci 2017; 55:80–7.

23. Alley JR. The clinical value of motion palpation as a diagnostic tool: A review. J Can Chiro Assoc 1983;27:97–100.

24. Holt K, Russell D, Cooperstein R, et al. Interexaminer reliability of seated motion palpation for the stiffest spinal site. J Manip Physiol Ther 2018;41:571–9.

25. Cooperstein R, Young M. The reliability of spinal motion palpation determination of the location of the stiffest spinal site is influenced by confidence ratings: a secondary analysis of three studies. Chiropr Man Ther 2016;24:50.

26. Cooperstein R, Young M, Haneline M. Interexaminer reliability of cervical motion palpation using continuous measures and rater confidence levels. J Can Chiropr Assoc 2013;57:156–64.

27. Libster AM, Lefler Y, Yaron-Jakoubovitch A, et al. Ataxia and the olivo-cerebellar module. Funct Neurol 2010;25:129–33.

28. Sandoz R. Some physical mechanisms and affects of spinal adjustments. Ann Swiss Chiropr Assoc 1976;6:91.

29. Scaringe JG, Faye LJ. Palpation: the art of manual assessment. In: Redwood D, Clevlan CI, editors. Fundamental of chiropractic. MIssouri: Mosby; 2003. p. 220.

30. Triano JJ, Budgell B, Bagnulo A, et al. Review of methods used by chiropractors to determine the site for applying manipulation. Chiropr Man Ther 2013;21:36.

31. Takatalo J, Ylinen J, Pienimäki T, et al. Intra- and inter-rater reliability of thoracic spine mobility and posture assessments in subjects with thoracic spine pain. BMC Muscoskel Disord 2020;21:529.

32. Gleberzon BJ, Cooperstein R, Good C, et al. Developing a standardized curriculum for teaching chiropractic technique. J Chiropr Educ 2021;35:249–57.

33. Bakkum B. Surface anatomy of the back and vertebral levels of clinically important structures. In: Cramer GDDS, editor. Clinical anatomy of the spine, spinal cord and ANS. 3rd edition. St. Louis, MO: Elsevier; 2014. p. 1–14.

34. Humphreys BK, Delahaye M, Peterson CK. An investigation into the validity of cervical spine motion palpation using subjects with congenital block vertebrae as a 'gold standard. BMC Muscoskel Disord 2004;5:19.

35. Zito G, Jull G, Story I. Clinical tests of musculoskeletal dysfunction in the diagnosis of cervicogenic headache. Man Ther 2006;11:118–29.

36. Cramer GD, Fournier JT, Henderson CN, et al. Degenerative changes following spinal fixation in a small animal model. J Manip Physiol Ther 2004;27:141–54.

37. Medina C, Jurek C, LoGiudice R. The role of acupuncture and manipulative therapy in canine rehabilitation. In: Zink C, Van Dyke JB, editors. *Canine Sports medicine and rehabilitation.* 2nd edition. Hoboken, NJ: Wiley Blackwell; 2018. p. 545–63.

38. Millis D. Responses of musculoskeletal tissues to disuse and remobilization. In: Millis D, Levine D, editors. Canine rehabilitation and physical therapy. 2nd edition. Philadelphia, PA: Elsevier; 2014. p. 92–153.

39. Nilsson N. The effects of spinal manipulation in the treatment of cervicogenic headaches. J Manip Physiol Ther 1997;20:326–30.

40. Arkuszewski Z. The efficacy of manual treatment in low back pain: a clinical trial. Manual Med 1986;2:68–71.

41. Rivera PL. Local, segmental, and suprasegmental influece of spinal manipulation, AAEP Proceedings, 64, 2018, 315-319.

42. Yate RTea. Effects of chiropractic treatment on blood pressure and anxiety: a randomized, controlled trial. J Manip Physiol Ther 1988;11:484–8.

43. ea Cassidy JD. The immediate effect of manipulation versus mobilization on pain and range of motion in the cervical spine: a randomized controlled trial. J Manip Physiol Ther 1992;15(9):570–5.

44. Pickar JG, Sung P, Kang Y, et al. Response of lumbar paraspinal muscles spindles is greater to spinal manipulative loading compared with slower loading under length control. Spine J 2007;7(5):583–95.

45. Cramer GD, Gregerson DM, Knudsen JT, et al. The effects of side-posture positioning and spinal adjusting on the lumbar Z joints: a randomized controlled trial with sixty-four subjects. Spine 2002;27:2459–66.

46. Cramer GD, Cambron J, Cantu JA, et al. Magnetic resonance imaging zygapophyseal joint space changes (gapping) in low back pain patients following spinal manipulation and side-posture positioning: a randomized controlled mechanisms trial with blinding. J Manipulative Physiol Therapeut 2013;36:203–17.

47. Cramer GD, Henderson CN, Little JW, et al. Zygapophyseal joint adhesions after induced hypomobility. J Manipulative Physiol Therapeut 2010;33:508–18.

48. Christiansen TL, Niazi IK, Holt K, et al. The effects of a single session of spinal manipulation on strength and cortical drive in athletes. Eur J Appl Physiol 2018;118:737–49.

49. Cramer G, Budgell B, Henderson C, et al. Basic science research related to chiropractic spinal adjusting: the state of the art and recommendations revisited. J Manipulative Physiol Therapeut 2006;29:726–61.

50. Cramer GD, Ross K, Pocius J, et al. Evaluating the relationship among cavitation, zygapophyseal joint gapping, and spinal manipulation: an exploratory case series. J Manipulative Physiol Therapeut 2011;34:2–14.

51. Webb AL, Collins P, Rassoulian H, et al. Synovial folds - a pain in the neck? Man Ther 2011;16:118–24.

52. Cramer GD, Bakkum BW. Microscopic anatomy of the zygapophysial joints, intervertebral discs, and other major tissues of the back. In: Cramer GD, Darby SA,

editors. Clinical anatomy of the spine, spinal cord, and ANS. 3rd Edition. MIssouri: Elsevier; 2014. p. 586–637.

53. Morningstar MW, Pettibon BR, Schlappi H, et al. Reflex control of the spine and posture: a review of the literature from a chiropractic perspective. Chiropr Osteopathy 2005;13:16.

54. Haussler K. The role of manual therapies in equine pain management. Vet Clin North Am Equine Pract 2010;26(23):579–601.

55. Haussler KK. Joint mobilization and manipulation for the equine athlete. Vet Clin North Am Equine Pract 2016;32:87–101.

56. Williams TF. The effect of cognitive behavioral therapy and chiropractic care on stress reduction. In: College of Social and Behavioral Sciences. Columbia, MD: Walden University; 2017.

57. Whelan TL, Dishman JD, Burke J, et al. The effect of chiropractic manipulation on salivary cortisol levels. J Manipulative Physiol Ther 2002;25:149–53.

58. Cramer SC, Sur M, Dobkin BH, et al. Harnessing neuroplasticity for clinical applications. Brain 2011;134:1591–609.

59. von Bernhardi R, Bernhardi LE, Eugenín J. What is neural plasticity? Adv Exp Med Biol 2017;1015:1–15.

60. Gomez-Alvarez CB, Moffat D, Back W, et al. Effect of chiropractic manipulation in the kinematics of back and limbs in horses with clinically diagnosed back problems. Equine Vet J 2008;40(42):153–9.

61. Cramer G. The clinical anatomy of spinal manipulative therapy. In: NUoH Sciences, editor. Healing Oasis wellness center - VSMT postgraduate certification Program. Sturtevant2016. 2021. p. 1–13.

62. Carnes DMT, Mullinger B, Froud R, et al. Adverse events and manual therapy: a systematic review. J Manual Ther 2010;15(4):355–63.

63. Oliphant D. Safety of spinal manipulation in the treatment of lumbar disk herniations: a systematic review and risk assessment. J Manip Physiol Therap 2004;27:197–210.

64. Church EW, Sieg EP, Zalatimo O, et al. Systematic review and meta-analysis of chiropractic care and cervical artery dissection: no evidence for causation. Cureus 2016;8:e498.

65. Kosloff TM ea. Chiropractic care and the risk of vertebrobasilar stroke: results of a case-control study in U.S. commercial and medicare advantage populations. Chiropr Man Ther 2015;23:19.

66. Smith DL, Cramer GD. Spinal manipulation is not an emerging risk factor for stroke nor is it major head/neck trauma. don't just read the abstract. Open Neurol J 2011;5:46–7.

67. Struewer J, Frangen TM, Ziring E, et al. Massive hematothorax after thoracic spinal manipulation for acute thoracolumbar pain. Orthop Rev 2013;5:e27.

68. Chung O. MRI confirmed cervical cord injury caused by spinal manipulation in a Chinese patient. Spinal Cord 2002;40:196–9.

69. Terrett A. Misuse of the literature by medical authors in discussing spinal manipulation therapy injury. Jour Manip Physiol Ther 1995;18:203–10.

70. ea Manga P. The effectiveness and cost-effectiveness of chiropractic management of low-back pain. Ontario: Ontario Ministry of Health; 1993.

71. Bigos SC. Clinical practice guidelines - number 14 - acute low back problems in adults. Rockville, MD: US Department of Health and Human Services, Public Health Service; Agency for Health Care Policy and Research; 1994.

72. Inoue M., Hasegawa A., Hosoi Y., et al., A current life table and causes of death for insured dogs in Japan, Prev Vet Med, 120, 2015, 210–218.

73. Kraus C, Pavard S, Promislow DEL, et al. The size-lefe span trade-off decomposed: why large dogs die young. Am Nat 2013;181:492–505.
74. Available at: https://www.aaha.org/aaha-guidelines/2023-aaha-senior-care-guidelines-for-dogs-and-cats/home/. Accessed March 14, 2023.
75. Seymour K., *Aging pets: senior, geriatric and what it all means to experts and readers, VetStreet*. Available at: https://www.vetstreet.com/our-pet-experts/aging-pets-senior-geriatric-and-what-it-all-means-to-experts-and-readers. Accessed March 14, 2023.
76. AHA) A.H.A., Euthanasia: making the decision fact sheet, Available at: http://www.americanhumane.org/fact-sheet/euthanasia-making-the-decision/. 2016, 2016. Accessed March 14, 2023.
77. Lorenz MD, Coates J, Kent M. Disorders of micturition. Handbook of veterinary neurology. 5th edition. St. Louis, MO: Elsevier - Saunders; 2011. p. 58–74.
78. Granger N, Olby NJ, Nout-Lomas YS. Bladder and bowel management in dogs with spinal cord injury. Front Vet Sci 2020;7:583342.
79. Thude TR. Chiropractic abnormalities of the lumbar spine significantly associated with urinary incontinence and retention in dogs. J Small Anim Pract 2015;56:693–7.
80. Rudinsky A. Top 5 Reasons for fecal house soiling in senior pets, Clinicians Brief. Accessed September 2016.
81. Acierno MJ, Labato MA. Canine incontinence. Vet Clin North Am Small Anim Pract 2019;49:125–40.
82. Heros R., Ciccone J., Kroopf L., et al., Essentials of Radiofrequency Ablation of the Spine and Joints, 2021, Sacroiliac Joint 135–170. ISBN: 978-3-030-78032-6
83. Henderson CN. The basis for spinal manipulation: chiropractic perspective of indications and theory. J Electromyogr Kinesiol 2012;22:632–42.
84. Schaub KI, Kelleners N, Schmidt MJ, et al. Three-dimensional kinematics of the pelvis and caudal lumbar spine in german shepherd dogs. Front Vet Sci 2021; 8:709966.
85. Wise R., Jones J., Werre S.,et al., The prevalence of sacroiliac joint CT and MRI findings is high in large breed dogs, *Vet Radiol Ultrasound*, 63 (6), 2022, 739–748.
86. American College of Physicians issues guideline for treating nonradicular low back pain, 2017, Available at: https://www.acponline.org/acp-newsroom/american-college-of-physicians-issues-guideline-for-treating-nonradicular-low-back-pain. Accessed March 14, 2023.
87. Cole C, Tully G. Reversal of Paraplegia Secondary to Intervertebral Disc Disease in 24 Canines with Vertebral Subluxation: A Retrospective Analysis of Outcomes Following Chiropractic. Annals of Vertebral Subluxation Research 2018;173–9.
88. Available at: ACVS. https://www.acvs.org/small-animal/cranial-cruciate-ligament-disease. Accessed March 17, 2023.
89. Adrian CP, Haussler KK, Kawcak C, et al. The role of muscle activation in cruciate disease. Vet Surg 2013;42:765–73.
90. Kirkby Shaw K, Alvarez L, Foster SA, et al. Fundamental principles of rehabilitation and musculoskeletal tissue healing. Vet Surg 2020;49:22–32.
91. Evans HE, De Lahunta A. Guide to the dissection of the dog. 7th edition. St. Louis, MO: Saunders/Elsevier; 2010.
92. Eberhardt L., Guevar J., Forterre F., The nerve root syndrome in small animals - a review focussing on pathophysilogy and therapy in the dog, *Tierarztl Prax*, 47, 2019, 344–357.
93. Suarez-Rodriguez V, Fede C, Pirri C, et al. Fascial innervation: a systematic review of the literature. Int J Mol Sci 2022;23(10):5674.

94. Schleip R, Jäger H, Klingler W. What is 'fascia'? A review of different nomenclatures. J Bodyw Mov Ther 2012;16:496–502.
95. Schultz R, Due T, Elbrond V. In: Anatomy trains in quadrupeds - initial investigations, Anatomy trains. 4th edition. Cambridge, MA: Elsevier; 2021. p. 347–54.
96. Zullo A, Mancini FP, Schleip R, et al. The interplay between fascia, skeletal muscle, nerves, adipose tissue, inflammation and mechanical stress in musculofascial regeneration. Journal Of Gerontology And Geriatrics 2017;65:271–83.
97. Cassidy JD ea. Risk of Vertebro-basilar stroke and chiropractic care: Results of a population based case-control and case-crossover study. Spine 2008;33: S176–83.
98. Cramer G. General characteristics of the spine. In: Cramer GDDS, editor. Clinical anatomy of the spine, spinal cord and ANS. 3rd edition. St. Louis, MO: Elsevier; 2014. p. 15–64.
99. Gkasdaris G, Kapetanakis S. Clinical anatomy and significance of the lumbar intervertebral foramen: a review. J Anat Soc India 2015;64:166–73.

Shockwave Therapy in Veterinary Rehabilitation

Carolina Medina, DVM, DACVSMR, CVA, CVPP

KEYWORDS

- Extracorporeal shockwave therapy • Shockwave • Shockwave therapy

KEY POINTS

- Extracorporeal shockwave therapy (ESWT) is a noninvasive treatment that involves the transcutaneous delivery of high-energy sound waves into tissue creating therapeutic effects.
- Musculoskeletal conditions that can benefit from ESWT include osteoarthritis, tendinopathies, fracture/bone healing, and wound healing.
- The most commonly used shockwave devices in small animals produce focused pressure pulses, which are electrohydraulic, electromagnetic, and piezoelectric.

HISTORY

Extracorporeal shockwave therapy (ESWT) initially received acceptance in the medical field in the 1980s for its use as lithotripsy treatment of urinary and renal calculi in people.[1] More recent human clinical trials have shown ESWT to be an effective treatment for lateral epicondylitis, plantar fasciitis, tendonitis, and fracture healing.[2–4] Numerous studies have shown that ESWT alleviated pain and lameness in horses with osteoarthritis and suspensory desmitis.[5–7] The preliminary canine studies followed a similar path to the human studies showing efficacy for the treatment of ureterolithiasis and nephrolithiasis.[8,9] Other canine studies have shown efficacy of ESWT for the treatment of fracture repair, osteoarthritis, supraspinatus calcifying tendinopathy, and patellar desmitis.[10–14] As evidence continues to grow, the use of ESWT in clinical veterinary practice is becoming more common.

MECHANISM OF ACTION

Shockwaves are nonlinear, high-pressure, high-velocity acoustic waves characterized by low tensile amplitude, short rise time to peak pressure, and a short duration (less than 10 milliseconds).[15] Shockwaves generate a single pulsed sound wave with a wide frequency range (16–20 MHz), high pressure amplitude (up to 100 MPa), and a short rise time (5–10 nanoseconds).[16] These single pulsed sound waves dissipate

Elanco Animal Health, 2500 Innovation Way, Greenfield, IN 46140, USA
E-mail address: carolina.medina@elancoah.com

Vet Clin Small Anim 53 (2023) 775–781
https://doi.org/10.1016/j.cvsm.2023.02.009
0195-5616/23/© 2023 Elsevier Inc. All rights reserved.
vetsmall.theclinics.com

mechanical energy at the interface of substances with different acoustic impedance. Shockwaves produce approximately 1000 times the pressure magnitude of ultrasound waves and deliver energy at a controlled focal volume. The mechanical energy transferred to tissues following ESWT causes various biological responses at the cellular level.[17] This mechanical stimulation of cells results in increased expression of cytokines and growth factors leading to decreased inflammation, neovascularization, and cellular proliferation.[1,18–20] Shockwaves transmit mechanical energy into tissues according to the tissue's acoustic impedance. Water and gel have low impedance allowing for best penetration of shockwaves into tissues. The sharp, rapid increase in pressure waves is followed by a negative pressure drop that leads to generation of cavitation bubbles with subsequent collapse; this leads to increased cellular permeability and production of free radicals followed by the generation of anti-inflammatory cytokines and growth factors to decrease pain and inflammation and remodel soft tissues.[21]

It is known that osteogenesis is induced by inhibition of osteoclasts. In bone augmentation, ESWT activates osteogenesis by osteoblast differentiation and then by increased proliferation.[22] ESWT has also been shown to inhibit cartilage degeneration and promote the rebuilding of subchondral bone in rat models with osteoarthritis. Computerized tomography (CT) scan findings of the study rats included increased bone density, bone volume, trabecular count, and trabecular strength, suggesting that ESWT promotes subchondral bone formation.[23] In addition, ESWT induces proliferation of periosteal cells.[24] In a rat study, shockwave therapy was applied to fracture repair sites using screws. CT showed an increase in bone density and increased stability.[25,26] It has been proven that ESWT speeds healing and increases quality of healing in soft tissues and bone, protects chondrocytes, disintegrates calcifications, and recruits stem cells to the treatment site.[2,20,27–29] The mechanism behind the pain-relieving effect of ESWT is thought to be due to increased serotonin activity in the dorsal horn and descending inhibition of pain signals.[1,4]

TYPES OF DEVICES

The most commonly used shockwave devices in small animals produce focused pressure pulses. The three types of focused shockwave generators are electrohydraulic, electromagnetic, and piezoelectric. Electrohydraulic devices have a spark plug in the trode that fires within a fluid medium, and they deliver focused, high-energy sound waves. Electromagnetic devices have induction coils that generate opposing magnetic fields that are focused on an acoustic lens, and they deliver low-pressure acoustic waves. Piezoelectric devices have crystals that expand and deform when stimulated by high-voltage electricity, and they deliver focused, low-energy ultrasonic waves. The depth of penetration of most focused shockwave devices is up to 12 cm.[21]

SCIENTIFIC EVIDENCE

Mueller *and colleagues* conducted a study to evaluate the effects of ESWT on the pelvic limb function of dogs suffering from coxofemoral osteoarthritis. Twenty-four client-owned dogs with coxofemoral osteoarthritis were investigated; eighteen of them received radial shockwave therapy and six were left untreated as controls. Force plate analysis on a treadmill was used to assess the dogs' pelvic limb function before treatment and 4 weeks after the last treatment. The ESWT dogs were reevaluated 3 and 6 months after treatment. In the ESWT dogs, differences between the ground reaction forces exerted by the right and left pelvic limbs disappeared 4 weeks after treatment, whereas in the control dogs, only the peak vertical force (PVF) distribution changed significantly. The significant improvement in the ESWT dogs was confirmed by changes in the symmetry indices. Significant improvements in vertical impulse (VI) and PVF were observed 3 months after treatment. Researchers concluded that ESWT is an effective treatment modality for dogs with coxofemoral osteoarthritis.[11]

Becker *and colleagues* performed a retrospective study, where they reviewed medical records of 15 dogs with shoulder lameness that failed previous conservative management. ESWT was administered every 3 to 4 weeks for a total of three treatments. Short-term, in-hospital subjective lameness evaluation revealed resolution of lameness in three of nine dogs and improved lameness in six of nine dogs available for evaluation 3 to 4 weeks following the last treatment. Long-term lameness score via telephone interview was either improved or normal in 7 of 11 dogs (64%). Researchers proposed that ESWT may result in improved function based on subjective patient evaluation and did not have any negative side effects in dogs with lameness attributable to instability, calcifying, and inflammatory conditions of the shoulder.[30]

Leeman *and colleagues* conducted a study using ESWT for shoulder tendinopathies to determine the association between shoulder lesion severity identified on ultrasonography or MRI and outcome and to compare the outcomes of dogs treated with ESWT with and without therapeutic exercises. Medical records of 29 dogs diagnosed with shoulder tendinopathies and treated with ESWT were reviewed, and 24 dogs were diagnosed with either unilateral biceps tendinopathy, or biceps tendinopathy and supraspinatus tendinopathy. Eighty-five percent of dogs had good or excellent outcomes determined by owner assessment 11 to 220 weeks after therapy. Outcomes were found to be better as tendon lesion severity increased ($P = .0497$), regardless if ESWT was performed with or without therapeutic exercise ($P = .92$). Researchers mentioned that ESWT should be considered a safe primary therapeutic option for canine shoulder tendinopathies and larger controlled prospective studies are needed to adequately assess these findings.[31]

A study was conducted to determine if shockwave therapy could promote neovascularization of the calcaneal tendon–bone junction. Eight mixed breed dogs received shockwave therapy on the right calcaneal bone–tendon junction. Biopsies were taken from the middle one-third of the calcaneal tendon–bone junction at 4 weeks and from the lateral one-third at 8 weeks, respectively, after shockwave application. Microscopic examination included the number of new capillaries and muscularized vessels, the presence and arrangements of myofibroblasts, and the changes in bone. New capillary and muscularized vessels were seen 4 and 8 weeks after shockwave, but none were seen in the control group before shockwave application. Myofibroblasts were not seen in the control group. Myofibroblasts with haphazard appearance and intermediate orientation fibers were seen in all study specimens obtained at 4 weeks and predominantly intermediate orientation myofibroblast fibers at 8 weeks. There were no changes in bone matrix, osteocyte activity, and vascularization within the bone. The results of the study suggest that shockwave-enhanced neovascularization at the bone–tendon junction in dogs.[32]

Kieves and colleagues evaluated the influence of ESWT on radiographic evidence of bone healing after tibial plateau leveling osteotomy (TPLO). Forty-two dogs (50 stifles) that underwent a TPLO were randomly assigned to receive either ESWT or sham. Treatments were delivered to the osteotomy site immediately postoperative, and a second treatment was done 2 weeks postoperative. Radiographs were evaluated by blinded radiologists 8 weeks postoperatively. Based on 5-point and 10-point bone healing scales, the mean healing scores were significantly greater in the ESWT group than the sham group. Researchers determined that ESWT led to more advanced bone healing after a TPLO.[33]

Gallagher and colleagues conducted a study to determine if ESWT after TPLO has a beneficial effect on patellar ligament inflammation assessed by thickening of the ligament and ligament fiber disruption. Thirty dogs that had TPLO had the affected stifle examined by radiographs and ultrasonography preoperative and 4, 6, and 8 weeks after TPLO. At 4 and 6 weeks, dogs in the treatment group were anesthetized and treated with ESWT. Patellar ligament thickness on a lateral radiographic projection was measured at a quarter, half, and three-quarter of the distance from origin to insertion. Ultrasound images were evaluated for patellar ligament disruption and periligamentous edema. A significant radiographic difference between groups was reached at 6 and 8 weeks postoperatively. No significant ultrasonographic differences were found. Researchers determined that ESWT decreases the radiographic signs of patellar ligament desmitis.[14]

Barnes *and colleagues* performed a randomized, prospective clinical trial to determine the influence of postoperative ESWT on hind limb use after TPLO. Sixteen client-owned dogs, 2 to 10 years old are weighing 18 to 75 kg. Dogs were randomly assigned to treatment cohorts, TPLO with ESWT (ESWT, $n = 9$) or TPLO without ESWT (control, $n = 7$). Treatment was instituted immediately postoperative and 2 weeks after surgery. Subjective pain, stifle goniometry, stifle circumference, peak vertical force (PVF), and VI were measured before surgery, before ESWT, and 2 and 8 weeks after surgery. Measures were compared between treatments at each time point and among time points for each treatment ($P < .05$). The PVF (5.5 ± 1.0 N/kg, mean $\pm$ SD) and VI (0.67 ± 0.14 N-s/kg) of surgically treated limbs in the ESWT cohort were higher 8 weeks after surgery compared with preoperative (3.8 ± 1.1 N/kg, $P < .0001$ and $.47 \pm 0.21$ N-s/kg, $P = .0012$, respectively) values. In the control cohort, PVF (2.9 ± 1.3 N/kg, $P = .0001$) and VI (0.33 ± 0.20 N-s/kg, $P = .0003$) 2 weeks after surgery and VI (0.42 ± 0.2 N-s/kg, $P = .0012$) 8 weeks after surgery were lower (4.59 ± 2.33 N/kg and 0.592 ± 0.35 N-s/kg, respectively) than before surgery. Other parameters did not differ between the groups. Researchers concluded that weight-bearing increased faster after TPLO in dogs treated with postoperative ESWT and that ESWT should be considered adjunctive therapy after TPLO.[34]

Barnes *and colleagues* conducted another study to compare optical values in the osteotomy gap created after a tibial tuberosity advancement (TTA) treated with autogenous cancellous bone graft, extracorporeal shock wave therapy, a combination of autogenous cancellous bone graft and extracorporeal shock wave therapy, and absence of both autogenous cancellous bone graft and extracorporeal shock wave therapy using densitometry. Dogs that were presented for surgical repair of a cranial cruciate ligament rupture were randomly assigned to one of four groups: TTA with autogenous cancellous bone graft (TTA-G), TTA with autogenous cancellous bone graft and extracorporeal shock wave therapy (TTA-GS), TTA with extracorporeal shock wave therapy (TTA-S), and TTA with no additional therapy (TTA-O). Mediolateral radiographs at 0, 4, and 8 weeks after surgery were evaluated to compare healing of the osteotomy gap via densitometry. An analysis of variance was used to compare the densitometric values between groups. At 4 weeks after surgery, a significant difference in osteotomy gap density was noted between TTA-GS (8.4 mm of aluminum equivalent [mmAleq]) and TTA-S (6.1 mmAleq) and between TTA-GS (8.4 mmAleq) and TTA-O (6.4 mmAleq). There were no significant differences noted between any groups at the 8-week reevaluation. There were no significant differences in the osteotomy gap density at 8 weeks after surgery regardless of the treatment modality used. The combination of autogenous cancellous bone graft and extracorporeal shock wave therapy may lead to increased radiographic density of the osteotomy gap in the first 4 weeks after surgery.[35]

SUMMARY

ESWT is a noninvasive treatment that involves the transcutaneous delivery of high-energy sound waves into tissue creating therapeutic effects. ESWT has been shown to increase expression of cytokines and growth factors leading to decreased inflammation, neovascularization, and cellular proliferation; activation of osteogenesis by osteoblast differentiation and then by increased proliferation; inhibition of cartilage degeneration and rebuilding of subchondral bone; and increased serotonin in the dorsal horn, and descending inhibition of pain signals. Musculoskeletal conditions that can benefit from ESWT include osteoarthritis, tendinopathies, fracture/bone healing, and wound healing.

CLINICS CARE POINTS

- Shave the fur and apply liberal amounts of ultrasound gel for proper penetration of the sound waves into tissue.
- Some devices and/or trodes that are quite powerful can cause some discomfort during the treatment, and therefore, sedation may be necessary.
- Treatments are typically performed, one to three treatments every 2 to 3 weeks, or as needed based on the clinical condition.

DISCLOSURE

The author has no conflicts of interest associated with this publication.

REFERENCES

1. Sems A, Dimeff R, Iannotti J. Extracorporeal shock wave therapy in the treatment of chronic tendinopathies. J Am Acad Orthop Surg 2006;14:95–204.
2. Gerdesmeyer L, Wagenpfeil S, Haake M, et al. Extracorporeal shock wave therapy for the treatment of chronic calcifying tendonitis of the rotator cuff: a randomized controlled trial. JAMA 2003;290:2573–80.
3. Haupt G, Haupt A, Ekkernkamp A, et al. Influence of shock waves on fracture healing. Urology 1992;39:529–32.
4. Rompe J, Rumler F, Hopf C, et al. Extracorporeal shock wave therapy for calcifying tendinitis of the shoulder. Clin Orthop Relat Res 1995;321:196–201.
5. Dahlberg J, McClure S, Evans R, et al. Force platform evaluation of lameness severity following extracorporeal shock wave therapy in horses with unilateral forelimb lameness. J Am Vet Med Assoc 2006;229:100–3.
6. Frisbie D, Kawcak C, McIlwraith C. Evaluation of the effect of extracorporeal shock wave treatment on experimentally induced osteoarthritis in middle carpal joints of horses. Am J Vet Res 2009;70:449–54.
7. Crowe O, Dyson S, Wright I, et al. Treatment of chronic or recurrent proximal suspensory desmitis using radial pressure wave therapy in the horse. Equine Vet J 2004;36:313–6.
8. Bailey G, Burk R. Dry extracorporeal shock wave lithotripsy for treatment of ureterolithiasis and nephrolithiasis in a dog. J Am Vet Med Assoc 1995;207(5):592–5.
9. Block G, Adams L, Widmer W, et al. Use of extracorporeal shock wave lithotripsy for the treatment of ureterolithiasis and nephrolithiasis in five dogs. J Am Vet Med Assoc 1996;208(4):531–6.

10. Johannes E, Kaulesar D, Matura E. High-energy shock waves for the treatment of nonunions: an experiment on dogs. J Surg Res 1994;57(2):246–52.
11. Mueller M, Bockstahler B, Skalicky M, et al. Effects of radial shockwave therapy on the limb function of dogs with hip osteoarthritis. Vet Rec 2007;160(22):762–5.
12. Dahlberg J, Fitch G, Evans R, et al. The evaluation of extracorporeal shockwave therapy in naturally occurring osteoarthritis of the stifle joint in dogs. Vet Comp Orthop Traumatol 2005;18(3):147–52.
13. Danova N, Muir P. Extracorporeal shock wave therapy for supraspinatus calcifying tendinopathy in two dogs. Vet Rec 2003;152(7):208–9.
14. Gallagher A, Cross A, Sepulveda G. The effect of shock wave therapy on patellar ligament desmitis after tibial plateau leveling osteotomy. Vet Surg 2012;41(4): 482–5.
15. Chung B, Wiley J. Extracorporeal shockwave therapy: A review. Sports Med 2002;32(13):851–65.
16. McClure S, Van Sickle D, White R. Effects of extracorporeal shockwave therapy on bone. Vet Surg 2004;33:40–8.
17. Niebaum K, McCauley L, Medina C. Rehabilitation Physical Modalities. In: Zink C, Van Dyke J, editors. Canine Sports medicine and Rehabilitation. 2nd edition. Hoboken, NJ: John Wiley & Sons, Inc; 2018. p. 136–76.
18. Wang F, Yang K, Chen R, et al. Extracorporeal shock wave promotes growth and differentiation of bone-marrow stromal cells towards osteoprogenitors associated with induction of TGF-beta1. J Bone Joint Surg Br 2002;84(3):457–61.
19. Wang C, Wang F, Yang K, Weng L, et al. Shock wave therapy induces neovascularization at the tendon-bone junction. A study in rabbits. J Orthop Res 2003; 21(6):984–9.
20. Wang C, Wang F, Huang C, et al. Treatment for osteonecrosis of the femoral head: comparison of extracorporeal shock waves with core decompression and bone-grafting. J Bone Joint Surg Am 2005;87(11):2380–7.
21. Alvarez L. Extracorporeal shockwave therapy for musculoskeletal pathologies. In: Duerr F, Elam L, editors. Veterinary Clinics, small animal practice, small animal Orthopedic medicine. Philadelphia, PA: Elsevier; 2022. p. 1033–42.
22. Wang F, Wang C, Chen Y, et al. Ras induction of superoxide activates ERK-dependent angiogenic transcription factor HIF-1 and VEGF-A expression in shock wave-stimulated osteoblasts. J Biol Chem 2004;279:10331–7.
23. Császár N, Angstman N, Milz S, et al. Radial shock wave devices generate cavitation. PLoS One 2015;10(10):e0140541.
24. Kearney C, Lee J, Padera R, et al. Extracorporeal shock wave-induced proliferation of periosteal cells. J Orthop Res 2011;29:1536–43.
25. van der Jagt O, van der Linden J, Schaden W, et al. Unfocused extracorporeal shock wave therapy as potential treatment for osteoporosis. J Orthop Res 2009;27:1528–33.
26. Koolen M, Kruyt M, Zadpoor A, et al. Optimization of screw fixation in rat bone with extracorporeal shock waves. J Orthop Res 2018;36:76–84.
27. Moretti B, Florenzo I, Notarnicola A, et al. Extracorporeal shock waves down-regulate the expression of interleukin-10 and tumor necrosis factor-alpha in osteoarthritic chondrocytes. BMC Musculoskelet Disord 2008;9:16.
28. Schaden W, Fischer A, Sailler A. Extracorporeal shock wave therapy of nonunion or delayed osseous union. Clin Orthop Relat Res 2001;387:90–4.
29. Aicher A, Heeschen C, Sasaki K, et al. Low-Energy Shock Wave for Enhancing Recruitment of Endothelial Progenitor Cells. Circulation 2006;114(25):2823–30.

30. Becker W, Kowaleski M, McCarthy R, et al. Extracorporeal Shockwave Therapy for Shoulder Lameness in Dogs. Am Anim Hosp Assoc 2015;51:15–9.
31. Leeman J, Shaw K, Mison M, et al. Extracorporeal shockwave therapy and therapeutic exercise for supraspinatus and biceps tendinopathies in 29 dogs. Vet Rec 2016 Ocy 15;179(15):385.
32. Wang C, Huang H, Pai C. Shockwave-enhanced neovascularization at the tendon-bone junction: an experiment in dogs. J Foot & Ankle Surgery 2002; 41(1):16–22.
33. Kieves N, Mackay C, Adducci K, et al. High energy focused shock wave therapy accelerates bone healing: A blinded, prospective, randomized, canine clinical trial. Vet Comp Orthop Traumatol 2015;28:425–32.
34. Barnes K, Faludi A, Takawira C, et al. Extracorporeal shock wave therapy improves short-term limb use after canine tibial plateau leveling osteotomy. Vet Surg 2019;48(8):1382–90.
35. Barnes K, Lanz O, Were S, et al. Comparison of autogenous cancellous bone grafting and extracorporeal shock wave therapy on osteotomy healing in the tibial tuberosity advancement procedure in dogs. Radiographic densitometric evaluation. Vet Comp Orthop Traumatol 2015;28(3):207–14.

Photobiomodulation (Therapeutic Lasers)

An Update and Review of Current Literature

Jessica Bunch, DVM, CCRT, CVA

KEYWORDS

- Photobiomodulation • Therapeutic laser • Laser therapy • Low-level laser therapy

KEY POINTS

- Photobiomodulation therapy (PBMT) is the use of red and near-infrared light to stimulate healing, relieve pain, and reduce inflammation.
- PBMT has the potential to be utilized for a variety of conditions in veterinary medicine, but limited studies exist for only a handful of conditions.
- There are currently no standardized treatment protocols for veterinary conditions and many different laser units available, resulting in an array of parameters used in research.
- Multiple parameters and patient factors can influence the effectiveness of PBMT and more clinical research with objective outcome measures is needed.

INTRODUCTION

Therapeutic laser usage in veterinary medicine continues to gain in popularity and momentum. As this modality advances and becomes a mainstay in many veterinary practices, we find that the terminology, research, and best practices continue to evolve and many gaps in our knowledge continue to exist. Laser is an acronym for *light amplification by stimulated emission of radiation*.[1,2] Laser is a focused and coherent beam of photons[3] that emit in an orderly fashion resulting in one wavelength (monochromatic) unlike ordinary light that showers us with a variety of wavelengths.[2] The principle of the laser dates to 1916 when Albert Einstein first described the theory of stimulated emission, but it was not until 1958 that Charles Townes and Arthur Schawlow wrote a paper on the proof of concept for creating one. In 1960, the first working laser was created by Theodore Maiman at Hughes Aircraft Company.[4] Experiments by Dr Endre Mester (Semmelweis Medical University, Hungary) in 1967 led to the discovery that low-level laser irradiation led to faster hair regrowth in mice compared with

Integrative Veterinary Medicine and Rehabilitation, College of Veterinary Medicine, Washington State University, 205 Ott Road, Pullman, WA 99164-7060, USA
E-mail address: jbunch@wsu.edu

Vet Clin Small Anim 53 (2023) 783–799
https://doi.org/10.1016/j.cvsm.2023.02.010
0195-5616/23/© 2023 Elsevier Inc. All rights reserved.

controls and coined the term "laser biostimulation". He later proceeded to stimulate wound healing in animal clinical trials.[1,3,5,6]

Laser Classifications

There are four major laser classifications (with a few subcategories) developed by American National Standards Institute and International Electrotechnical Institute. The primary basis for the classifications is the potential to cause damage to the eye or skin. They are based on energy or power, wavelengths, exposure duration, and the cross-sectional area of the laser beam at the point of interest.[7] The most common classes of lasers currently used for photobiomodulation in human and veterinary medicine are Class 3 B and Class 4, however, there is a growing use of Classes 1 and 2 as well as LEDs and other forms of light therapy. Basic descriptions for the classifications are in **Table 1**.

Definitions/Terminology

Many different names have been utilized and some continue to be used when discussing laser biostimulation leading to a lack of consistency in the literature and in practice. These include low-level laser therapy (LLLT), cold laser, high-intensity laser therapy, soft laser, Class 3b laser, therapy laser, Class 4 laser, photobiostimulation, and photobiomodulation.[1,5] LLLT has been commonly used in many studies, but many terms are vague and other forms of light therapy besides laser (such as LEDs) have been shown to stimulate healing. In 2016, the term photobiomodulation was added as a Medical Search Heading at the National Library of Medicine[5,8] and has been increasingly used in both human and veterinary medicine. Photobiomodulation therapy (PBMT) is the use of red and near-infrared light to stimulate healing, relieve pain and reduce inflammation.[8,9]

To better understand photobiomodulation, we need to become familiar with some of the more common terms and parameter definitions (**Table 2**).

Wavelengths

The electromagnetic spectrum runs from short gamma rays to very long radio waves and includes visible and invisible light. As previously mentioned, the wavelength is a major factor in determining the absorption and depth of penetration of a laser beam.[1] Ultraviolet light (100–400 nm) is absorbed by primarily melanin, proteins, and nucleic acid. Visible light (400–760 nm) is scattered and absorbed with absorption primarily in melanin, hemoglobin, and myoglobin and is therefore more suited for superficial conditions. With near-infrared light (760–1200 nm), photons are scattered but absorbed by a variety of chromophores and are better for deeper tissues. Above 1400 nm results in the absorption almost entirely of water.[10]

Mechanisms of Actions

Numerous studies are showing the beneficial effects of photobiomodulation and although some mechanisms of actions have been demonstrated at least in vitro, many are still not entirely understood. Many of the mechanisms center around the modulation of the inflammatory response and increasing cellular respiratory and metabolic rates. There are multiple proposed mechanisms of action involved in PBMT but the three major players are adenosine triphosphate (ATP), nitric oxide (NO), and reactive oxygen species (ROS).[1,5,8]

The photons being emitted from our therapeutic lasers are being absorbed by a variety of photo acceptors called chromophores.[5] One of the primary chromophores to be simulated is cytochrome c oxidase (CcO) also known as Complex IV in the

Table 1
Basic description for the classifications of lasers[7]

Class 1	Class 2	Class 3	Class 4
• no damage to eye/skin at any level • ex: laser printers	• limited to 1 mw CW or more if emission time is < 25 s or if the light is not spatially coherent • ex: retail scanners	• 5 mw to 500 mw • Can be an optical hazard with direct or reflected viewing of the beam. Protected eyewear should be worn when operating	• 500 mw • Potential to cause damage to the eye and skin • Protective eyewear must be worn when operating. • Includes therapeutic, surgical, and even industrial lasers

mitochondria and is the last enzyme in the electron transport chain.[5,8] When exposed to light at the appropriate wavelengths (red and infrared spectrum, approximately 500–1100 nm),[1,10] photons dissociate inhibiting nitric oxide bound to CcO, leading to an increase in the electron transport chain, mitochondrial membrane potential, and an increase in ATP production.[1] Increased ATP production may result in the following.

- An increase in energy to be utilized for a variety of reparative tasks[1]
- Increased cellular signaling[5]
- Increased intracellular calcium[5]
- May react as a neurotransmitter when released by nerve cells[5]

As previously mentioned, CcO may have nitric oxide bound to it, especially when under oxidative stress.[5] Photo-dissociation results in an increase in circulating nitric oxide.[1,5,10] The effects of increased nitric oxide are multiple including

- Increased metabolic turnover and normalization of cellular respiration[1,5]
- Mediation of vasodilation via relaxation of the endothelial cells[1,5]
- Increased angiogenesis[1,5]
- Modulation of the inflammatory and immune responses.[1,5]

Acceleration of the electron transport chain does result in the release of ROS. When laser is used at appropriate low levels, the levels of ROS produced are below damaging levels and can be beneficial.[1] Low levels of ROS can

- Activate antioxidant enzymes[1,5]
- Have stimulatory and signaling effects on cellular growth[1,5]
- Enhance stem cell differentiation[1,5]

However, in high levels of oxidative stress and chronic inflammatory processes, we see elevated levels of ROS. In these cases, photobiomodulation has been found to decrease ROS as well as decrease the expression and release of pro-inflammatory cytokines.[5,9,11]

For many of the uses of photobiomodulation in veterinary medicine, there are proposed and demonstrated mechanisms for the benefits seen in vitro and in laboratory animal models. The primary areas of research thus far have revolved around the role of PBMT for pain, musculoskeletal conditions, neurologic disease and dysfunction, and wound healing. **Table 3** summarizes some of these mechanisms.

Table 2
Common terms and parameter definitions used with photobiomodulation[1,3,5,9]

Term	Abbreviation	Definition
Chromophore		A molecule that absorbs photons at certain wavelengths (photo acceptor). For example, melanin, hemoglobin, porphyrins, CcO (cytochrome C oxidase)
Wavelength	Measured in nanometers (nm)	The distance between two successive points in a wave that is characterized by the same phase of oscillation. Different wavelengths of visible light are perceived by the eye as different colors. The wavelength of a laser determines its absorption properties and depth of penetration.
Joule	J	Unit of energy or work. The total number of joules delivered per session is equal to the total energy emitted per session.
Watt	W	The SI unit of power, equivalent to 1 J/s.
Dose/Fluence	J/cm^2	A measure of the amount of energy delivered to the surface of the target tissue.
Power	W	The rate at which energy is emitted. An expression of energy over time vs the total amount delivered. Expressed in watts (1 W = 1 J/s).
Irradiance/Power Density	W/cm^2	Density of radiation/power on a given surface.
Continuous Wave	CW	Emission of radiant energy in a constant intensity at a specific power.
Frequency	Measured in hertz (Hz)	The number of light waves passing a fixed point in a specific time interval (the number of cycles per second). Eg, 1 Hz = one light wave passed per second. Referred to as pulse rate/pulsing.
Spot Size		The radius of the laser beam. The width of the laser beam at the surface of the tissue being treated.

Research and reviews in human medicine

Photobiomodulation research has continued to grow over the last several decades with most studies coming from in vitro, human, and laboratory animal models. Various systematic reviews and meta-analyses have been undertaken as well as Cochrane

Table 3
A summary of proposed and demonstrated mechanisms for photobiomodulation[1,9–12]

Pain	• Decrease in bradykinins, pro-inflammatory interleukins, cytokines, and other inflammatory mediators[1,5] • Increase in the pain threshold via inhibition of Aδ and C fibers[1,2,10] • Raises cell action potential of nerves[1,10] • Increased levels of endorphins and activation of endogenous opioids[1,5,10,11] • Increased inhibitory neurotransmitters[1] • Increased serotonin[1,10]
Musculoskeletal	• Decrease in bradykinins, COX-2 production, and inflammatory cells in joint fluid[1] • Decrease in pro-inflammatory mediators in the joint and tendons[1] • Increased fibroblast proliferation and collagen synthesis[1,5] • Increased collagen fibril size, tensile strength, and improved fiber organization[1] • Increased myofibril formation and maturation[1] • Decreased muscle fatigue, lactate, and delayed muscle-onset soreness[1,8] • Decreased muscle inflammatory markers[1] • Accelerated bone healing and osteoblast proliferation[1]
Neurologic	• Inhibition of ROS and pro-inflammatory cytokines in the spinal cord[1] • Modulates release of IL-6 and IL-8 from the annulus fibrosis[1] • Promotion of axonal regeneration[1,10] • Decreased degeneration of peripheral nerve motor neurons in spinal cord[1] • Increased neurite fiber sprouting and Schwann cell proliferation[1,12] • Decreased scar formation[1] • Increased ATP and improved brain blood flow[12] • Reduction of brain beta-amyloid load and deposition[12] • Stimulation of brain-derived neurotrophic factor (BDNF)[12] • Reduction of neuroinflammation and oxidative injury[12]
Wounds	• Upregulated production and expression of growth factors[1,10] • Increased stem cells and progenitor cells[5] • Increased ATP[1,5] • Increased angiogenesis and vasodilation via increased NO[1,5,10] • Enhanced cellular differentiation, collagen deposition, and organization[1]

reviews regarding LLLT use for a variety of conditions. Cochrane reviews thus far support that LLLT may be beneficial for the following.

- Short-term relief of pain and stiffness for rheumatoid arthritis[13]
- Reduction in severity of chemotherapy-induced mucositis[14]
- Treatment of pain following orthodontic treatments[15]
- Short-term benefits for rotator cuff injuries[16]
- Decreased pain and improved function for frozen shoulder (adhesive capsulitis)[17]

Results for carpal tunnel syndrome[18] and non-specific low-back pain[19] had low quality, mixed results and insufficient evidence to support LLLT. It is important to note that for these reviews, many are outdated, a limited number of studies were reviewed, and many conditions are not represented. The overwhelming majority of criticism by each Cochrane review was the lack of quality of study design, lack of blinding and potential high bias, and no consistency in reporting of parameters and application techniques.

Additional systematic reviews with meta-analysis have also produced mixed results when it comes to proof of efficacy for PBMT. A 2018 systematic review by Rosso and colleagues[20] evaluated 26 articles looking at PBMT effects on peripheral nerve regeneration. Beneficial effects on recovery of nerve lesions were seen, especially when related to faster regeneration and functional improvement. Huang and colleagues[21] (2015) reviewed seven randomized clinical trials and concluded that LLLT was effective for relieving chronic low back pain but there was a lack of evidence supporting an improvement in function. Huang and colleagues[22] (2015) also performed a systematic review looking at LLLT's role in knee osteoarthritis (OA) and concluded that the evidence from nine trials did not support its effectiveness. There have also been two separate meta-analyses and systematic reviews that are more heterogenetic in nature. Tumilty and colleagues[23] reviewed 25 trials utilizing LLLT for various tendinopathies and found half of the studies showed positive effects whereas the other half were inconclusive or had no effect. In 2017, Clijsen and colleagues[24] concluded after reviewing 18 studies of various musculoskeletal disorders ranging from OA to back pain to tendinopathies, that LLLT is an effective modality to decrease pain in a variety of disorders especially when the dosages used are within the range of the recommendations by World Association of Photobiomodulation Therapy.

Veterinary research/clinical trials

In the last 10 years, there has been growth in veterinary medicine clinical trials especially in complementary modalities, in part, due to the expansion of physical rehabilitation and sports medicine in the veterinary field and the need for non-pharmaceutical therapies in addressing pain. Photobiomodulation has rapidly grown in popularity not just in specialty rehabilitation practices but also in general companion animal practice. In addition to clinical trials for treatment of various conditions in veterinary medicine, there have been several studies investigating some of the application factors that could affect the effectiveness of PBMT. A 2020 investigation by Hochman-Elam and colleagues examined the effects of laser power, wavelength, coat color, and coat length on tissue penetration using PBMT in healthy dogs. This study concluded that hair length and coat color did affect tissue penetration with longer and darker coats having less penetration. Given what we know about melanin's absorption properties through a large portion of our therapeutic light spectrum, this is not surprising regarding coat color and adjustments to power and/or considering shaving may be indicated for optimal results. A limitation of this study was that the penetration amount was measured through two layers of skin, subcutaneous tissues, and hair. The amount which affected the outcomes could not be estimated, therefore, more studies are warranted.[25] In 2019, Piao and colleagues[26] demonstrated that transcutaneous photobiomodulation light could penetrate the spinal cord of a cadaver dog model after receiving a hemilaminectomy. However, it was shown that on-contact with skin increased transmission by 67% compared with non-contact.

For the remainder of this article, we will examine what has been reported in clinical trials thus far relating to several conditions with a primary focus on neurologic and musculoskeletal applications. A summary of findings for the discussed trials can be found in **Table 4**.

Osteoarthritis

OA is one of the most common musculoskeletal disorders treated in companion animals, especially in our aging population. It is estimated that up to 20% of dogs over 1 year of age[27] and 40% of cats of any age,[28] exhibit clinical signs of OA. Treatment of this condition often involves a multi-modal approach which is increasingly involving photobiomodulation. A 2020 qualitative survey of Missouri veterinarians by Barger and colleagues, found 43% of respondents utilized LLLT units in the treatment of OA, and

Table 4
General information of referenced veterinary clinical studies (excluding dermatologic-related studies)[a]

Study	Type	n	Condition treated and Treatment length	Parameters	Outcomes
Alves et al,[30] 2022	DB-RCT[b]	40	Bilateral hip OA[c] 3 sessions/week 1 2 sessions/week 2 1 session/week 3	Class IV; 980 nm- dark coat 980/808 blend light/ medium coats 6.5-8 W; 4.5-8.2 W/cm² 14.3-19.5 J/cm² In-contact scanning grid pattern Sham PBMT: laser not turned on	Improvement in most CMI[d] scores by day +8 up to Day +30. Improved ROM by day +15 up to Day +90 vs meloxicam for control
de Oliveira Reusing et al,[31] 2021	DB-RCT	32	Hip dysplasia 2x/week x 2 months	904 nm; 2000 Hz; 20–50 mW 285.7 mW/cm²; 4–6 J Shaved point-to-point	Decreased pain scores both PBMT groups. Improved QOL[e], locomotion, and ROM[f] in PBMT w/hydro group and hydro alone group
Looney et al,[32] 2018	DB-RCT	20	Elbow OA 2x/week for 3 weeks 1x/week for 3 weeks	Class IV 980 nm and 650 nm (aiming beam) CW[g]; 10–20 J/cm² 5–12 W; 1–2.4 W/cm² Scanning grid method, not shaved Off contact < ½ cm Sham: 650 nm	Improved lameness scores, decreased pain scores, and reduction in NSAID use in 9/11 dogs
Barale et al,[33] 2019	Retrospective	17	OA multiple joints and associated muscles (hips, elbows, stifle, LS) Weekly x 6 weeks	808 nm; 1000 mW; 1 W/cm²; 500–1000 Hz joints; 3000–5000 Hz- muscles 4.2–5 J/cm² CW and PW[h] direct contact	CBPI[i] and VAS[j] scores decreased overtime. Reduction in analgesics in 13/17 dogs.

(continued on next page)

Table 4
(continued)

Study	Type	n	Condition treated and Treatment length	Parameters	Outcomes
Kennedy et al,[36] 2018	DB-RCT	12	Post-op TPLO Before and after surgery, 6, 12, 24, 36, 48, 60, 72, 84, and 96 h post-op At home: every other day x 4 weeks	Class 2 dual probe 4 x 5 mw diodes 635 nm; shaved 2.25 J/cm² in hospital 1.5 J/cm² at home Sham: replaced diodes w/ red LED light bulbs in unit	No significant differences between treatment and control.
Renwick et al,[37] 2017	DB-RCT	95	Post-op TPLO Day of surgery and 2 days post-op optional 4th (10–14 days post-op)	Class IV; shaved 660 nm (100 mW), 800, 905, 970 nm (max 15 W CW, 20 W PW) Sham: 660 nm; 4 mW	Greater improvement in gait section of adjusted COI*. No other improvements in CMIs or bone healing.
Rogatko et al,[38] 2017	DB-RCT	27	Pre-op TPLO 1 session pre-op	Class IV 800 nm and 970 nm; CW and PW 6 W; 3.5 J/cm² Shaved Sham: same unit turned off	Significant difference in PBMT group at 8 weeks post-op on PVF‡; greater proportion healed at 8 weeks (5/8 vs 3/12) but not significant
Draper et al,[39] 2012	Prospective (not blinded)	36	Post-op hemilaminectomy Daily x 5 days	810 nm 5 x 200 mW cluster array (1W) 25 W/cm² 2–8 J/cm²	PBMT group median time to ambulation 3–5 days vs 14 days for control

Bennaim et al,[40] 2017	DB-RCT	32	Post-op hemilaminectomy 6 treatments (PBMT) ± Rehab	Treatment group: 810 nm 1-W (5 × 20 mW) cluster probe Peak power 227 mW; 2.5 Hz: 88% duty cycle; 5.5 W/cm²; 12 J; 329.7 J/cm²; Sham: 660 nm; 4 × 6 mW; 30 W/cm²	No significant differences for any treatment groups
Bruno et al,[41] 2020	Retrospective	24	Post-op hemilaminectomy Minimum: 5 days/week x 2 weeks Rehab ± PBMT	808 nm CW, 905 nm PW 1.2 W, peak power 75 W 50% duty cycle; 18 Hz; 4 J/cm² Shaved, in contact, perilesional	No significant difference in time to ambulation but shorter mean time to ambulation in laser group
Miller et al,[42] 2020	Retrospective	20	Degenerative myelopathy PBMT + rehab 1-2x/week	Protocol A: 904 nm; 0.5 W; 0.5 W/cm², 8 J/point; point-to-point grid x 20 pts Protocol B: 980 nm; 6–12 W; 1.2–2.4 W/cm²; 14–21 J/cm²; moving grid pattern Both protocols: in contact, not shaved	Mean time of onset clinical signs and time of NAPᵐ and euthanasia in protocol B group. Mean time between start of treatment and times of euthanasia significantly longer in Protocol B

(continued on next page)

Table 4
(continued)

Study	Type	n	Condition treated and Treatment length	Parameters	Outcomes
Alves et al,[49] 2022	DB-RCT	30	Idiopathic chronic large bowel diarrhea 3 sessions/week 1 2 sessions/week 2 1 session/week 3	980/808 nm blend (80% 980 nm/20% 808 nm) 12 W: 1.92 W/cm^2(980 nm) 0.48 W/cm^2 (808 nm); 6.9 J/cm^2(980 nm) 1.7 J/cm^2 (808 nm); continuous grid pattern Off contact Sham: laser turned off	Improved fecal and CIBDAI[n] scores, decreased frequency of diarrhea, increased BW[o] and BCS[p] vs control (psyllium)

[a] Disclaimer: All information presented in this table is as reported in each study and a brief description. Some parameters may be incomplete or lacking. Please refer to each study for more information.
[b] DB-RCT, double-blinded, randomized clinical trial.
[c] OA, osteoarthritis.
[d] CMI, clinical metrology instruments.
[e] QOL, quality of life.
[f] ROM, range of motion.
[g] CW, continuous wave.
[h] PW, pulsed wave.
[i] CBPI, canine brief pain inventory.
[j] VAS, visual analog scale.
[k] COI, Canine Orthopedic Index.
[l] PVF, peak vertical force.
[m] NAP, non-ambulatory paresis/paralysis.
[n] CIBDAI, canine inflammatory bowel disease index.
[o] BW, body weight.
[p] BCS, body condition score.

of those who did not have a unit, 20% referred their patients for laser therapy. The estimated annual impact for treating one arthritic joint in Missouri was $6.2 million/year.[29]

There is growing evidence to support the use of PBMT in dogs with elbow and/or hip OA. A recent trial by Alves and colleagues[30] demonstrated PBMT was more effective for decreasing pain and improving clinical findings in working dogs with bilateral coxofemoral OA versus meloxicam. The effects of hydrotherapy and LLLT in canine hip dysplasia were investigated in a 2021 clinical study by de Oliveira Reusing and colleagues[31] They found that both therapies (alone or together) decreased chronic pain indices and improved quality of life, and hydrotherapy alone or with laser improved pain scores, joint range of motion, and thigh circumference. Regarding elbow OA, Looney and colleagues[32] found improvement in lameness scores, decreased pain scores, and decreased requirement for NSAIDs in a PBMT-treated group versus a sham-treated group. Lastly, a retrospective study by Barale and colleagues reviewed findings in 17 dogs with OA (various locations) treated with LLLT. They found a decrease in pain scores, an increase in function as well as a decreased need for analgesics at week 2 in 13/17 dogs.[33]

Cranial cruciate ligament disease

Cranial cruciate ligament disease (CCLD) is a very common affliction in our canine population, especially in large-breed dogs. One of the most common surgical corrections is the tibial plateau leveling osteotomy (TPLO). There have been three studies to date looking at the use of photobiomodulation for improving post-operative recovery in dogs, but no studies for its possible role in conservative management. Recently Alvarez and colleagues performed a systematic review of post-operative rehabilitation interventions after cranial cruciate ligament surgery in dogs. They concluded that current studies supported therapeutic exercise and cold compression therapy in improving clinical outcomes post-CCL surgery but not photobiomodulation.[34]

A 2017 systematic review by Bayat and colleagues[35] found that 75 out of 76 studies utilizing LLLT showed positive effects on fractures in animal models including acceleration and stimulation of fracture healing as well as callus formation. However, a 2018 Kennedy and colleagues[36] clinical trial in post-operative TPLO dogs showed no beneficial effects when utilizing a Class II laser on bone healing or pain reduction. Similarly, the 2017 Renwick study utilizing a Class IV laser for three treatments postoperatively also did not show improved bone healing and the only improved clinical metrology outcome was a greater improvement in the gait section of the adjusted Canine Orthopedic Index.[37] It is interesting to note that a study by Rogatko and colleagues investigating the effects of a single pre-operative LLLT treatment did not find a statistical difference in bone healing but a greater proportion of the treated dogs were healed at 8 weeks post-op. They also found a significant difference in peak vertical force in the treatment group at 8 weeks versus the sham group, however, no other significant changes were detected.[38]

Neurologic conditions

As we have seen in some human and rodent models, PBMT is a potential adjunctive therapy for back pain and peripheral nerve regeneration. Therefore, it is not difficult to attempt to translate this to canine models as well. Several studies have investigated the use of LLLT for post-operative recovery following hemi-laminectomies to treat intervertebral disc extrusion. These studies have thus far proven to have mixed results. One of the first promising studies was the 2012 Draper and colleagues' prospective trial of 36 dogs of which half were treated once daily for 5 days. The median time to ambulation was 3.5 days in the treatment group compared with 14 days in the control group. However, the limitations of this study included lack of blinding and incomplete randomization.[39] In contrast, a 2017 study by Bennaim and colleagues[40] evaluated the effects of PBMT and rehabilitation on the early post-operative recovery of dogs after hemi-laminectomy and found no difference between any treatment group and the control group. Lastly, a retrospective study by Bruno and colleagues[41] in 2020 reviewed dogs which had received perilesional PBMT in addition to rehabilitation versus rehabilitation alone post-operatively and found that although there was no statistical significance in time to regain ambulation between groups, there was a tendency for a shorter mean time in the laser group.

Beyond intervertebral disc disease, one retrospective observational study investigated the possible effects of photobiomodulation in the treatment of canine degenerative myelopathy in combination with physical rehabilitation. This 2020 study by Miller and colleagues found that the time between symptom onset and non-ambulatory paresis/paralysis (NAP) and/or euthanasia was lengthened for dogs treated with PBMT at higher irradiance and fluence versus dogs receiving a lower irradiance and fluence as well as published historical data. This was also true regarding the start of treatment and development of NAP and/or euthanasia in the higher dose group. It should also be noted that both lasers had several varying parameters (see **Table 4**). This suggests that PBMT, in addition to rehabilitation and with certain parameters, may slow disease progression thereby improving survival times.[42]

Other conditions

Photobiomodulation has the potential to be beneficial for a multitude of other conditions, many of which are outside the scope of this summary or have not yet been investigated. A few conditions to note are regarding photobiomodulation's effects on various skin conditions and wounds as well as a recent investigation into its use for chronic idiopathic large-bowel diarrhea.

Several small clinical trials in dogs have demonstrated the beneficial effects of PBMT in the healing of chronic wounds,[43] incisional healing after hemilaminectomies,[44] and decreasing bacterial counts in contaminated wounds.[45] There have been many lab animal and in vitro studies investigating the effects of PBMT on skin healing including a study by Gagnon and colleagues[20] that demonstrated in vitro that there was increased cellular migration and proliferation of cells in a canine healing skin model at 2 J/cm^2 versus non-irradiated cells, yet higher doses of 6 J/cm^2 decreased cellular migration and proliferation demonstrating what is called a biphasic dose response or Arndt-Schultz law. PBMT has also been shown to be beneficial for hair regrowth as demonstrated by Mester's original studies. A 2015 study by Olivieri and colleagues[46] demonstrated that six out of seven dogs with non-inflammatory alopecia had greatly improved hair growth when treated with photobiomodulation and one dog showed some improvement. There was also increased hair growth in the study by Schendeker and colleagues[47] when PBTM was used to treat acral lick dermatitis, however, there was no significant difference in the amount of licking, lesion size, or thickness. PBMT has also failed to improve the severity or pruritis score of dogs with pedal dermatitis secondary to canine atopic dermatitis. It should be noted that in this study, each dog was used as its own control and a lower pruritis score occurred for both the treated and non-treated foot. This is likely from a placebo effect but could also be due to possible systemic effects of PBMT therapy affecting both feet.[48]

One newly investigated area is utilizing PBMT's effects to aid in the treatment of idiopathic chronic large-bowel diarrhea. The recent 2022 study by Alves and colleagues explored using PBMT to aid in conservative management of large-bowel diarrhea in working dogs versus psyllium. Improvement was seen in multiple outcomes for the treatment group including an improvement in canine inflammatory bowel disease index, improved fecal scores, decreased frequency of episodes, increased body condition score, and increase body weight. This initial study holds promise that PBMT could serve as an adjunctive treatment modality in decreasing the clinical signs of this condition which can be seen in high-level working and competition dogs.[49]

DISCUSSION

The research thus far in veterinary medicine is growing stronger to support the adjunctive use of photobiomodulation for OA, wounds, and hair regrowth. There is early evidence for its use in degenerative myelopathy when used in conjunction with physical rehabilitation and idiopathic chronic large-bowel diarrhea. There have been several studies looking at the use of PBMT for enhancing recovery in post-operative hemilaminectomies patients, but thus far, the results have been mixed. Regarding postoperative orthopedic surgeries, PBMT use post-TPLO surgery has failed to yield strong evidence in enhancing recovery. Many conditions that are commonly treated in general practice, such as conservative management of CCLD and intervertebral disc disease, edema from trauma, soft tissue injuries such as tendinopathies, injury recovery, and more, have yet to be investigated. There are also proposed uses for a variety of other conditions and one recent publication by Dewey and colleagues[12] reviews the mechanisms of PBMT and its potential applications for transcranial use to treat canine cognitive dysfunction. It should be noted that most studies, including those that failed to yield positive results, did not show any negative or detrimental effects of PBMT when used within suggested and accepted parameters.

Many advances in photobiomodulation therapy have been made in the veterinary field in the last decade, however, more work is needed. Most of these clinical trials have had small sample sizes and varying levels of potential bias. Additionally, there are multiple parameters that affect beam penetration, divergence, and dose delivery to the target tissue. Consistency in parameter reporting is essential to draw more definitive conclusions regarding protocols used and to help create more standardization of treatment. Finally, there is an increased need for double-blinded, randomized, placebo-controlled clinical trials utilizing objective outcome measures in areas already studied as well as the multitude of other conditions that anecdotally have benefited from PBMT.

SUMMARY

Photobiomodulation therapy, also commonly referred to as LLLT, is a modality commonly used in companion animal physical rehabilitation as well as in general practice. Its role in decreasing inflammation, decreasing pain, and speeding reparative processes, is becoming more understood, accepted, and proven with increasing research. The ease of use by support staff, patient acceptance, and client awareness also lend to the popularity and demand for this therapy option. This modality has embedded itself as a non-invasive, non-pharmaceutical therapeutic adjunctive option for a wide variety of pathologies and has the promise to continue to grow in our field.

CLINICS CARE POINTS

- PBMT is the use of red and near-infrared light to stimulate healing, relieve pain and reduce inflammation.
- Multiple parameters affect the depth of penetration of photons and effects on the target tissue including wavelength, fluence, and irradiance.

- Application techniques and other factors may also affect penetration and absorption including contact versus non-contact, haired versus shaved, coat color, and coat length.
- PBMT has the potential to be utilized for a variety of conditions with stronger research to support some conditions over others such as OA.
- Most veterinary studies have shown PBMT to be safe when used with recommended parameters.
- More rigorous studies with objective outcome measures are needed for many conditions as well as optimizing best practices and treatment parameters.

DISCLOSURE

The author has nothing to disclose.

REFERENCES

1. Hochman L. Photobiomodulation therapy in veterinary medicine: a review. Top Companion Anim Med 2018;33(3):83–8.
2. Heiskanen V, Hamblin MR. Photobiomodulation: lasers vs. light emitting diodes? Photobiol Sci 2018;17(8):1003–17.
3. Zein R, Selting W, Hamblin MR. Review of light parameters and photobiomodulation efficacy: dive into complexity. J Biomed Opt 2018;23(12):1–17.
4. Riegel RJ. The history of laser therapy. In: Laser therapy in veterinary medicine. John Wiley & Sons, Inc; 2017. p. 1–6.
5. Anders JJ, Ketz AK, Wu X. Basic principles of photobiomodulation and its effects at the cellular, tissue, and system levels. In: Laser therapy in veterinary medicine. John Wiley & Sons, Inc; 2017. p. 36–51.
6. Anders JJ, Lanzafame RJ, Arany PR. Low-level light/laser therapy versus photobiomodulation therapy. Photomed Laser Surg 2015;33(4):183.
7. Bartels KE. Therapy laser safety. In: Laser therapy in veterinary medicine. John Wiley & Sons, Inc; 2017. p. 29–35.
8. Hamblin MR. Mechanisms and applications of the anti-inflammatory effects of photobiomodulation. AIMS Biophysics 2017;4(3):337–61.
9. Smith JJ. General principles of laser therapy. In: Laser therapy in veterinary medicine. John Wiley & Sons, Inc; 2017. p. 53–66.
10. Pryor B, Millis DL. Therapeutic laser in veterinary medicine. Vet Clin North Am Small Anim Pract 2015;45(1):45–56.
11. Pereira FC, Parisi JR, Maglioni CB, et al. Antinociceptive effects of low-level laser therapy at 3 and 8 j/cm2 in a rat model of postoperative pain: possible role of endogenous Opioids. Lasers Surg Med 2017;49(9):844–51.
12. Dewey CW, Brunke MW, Sakovitch K. Transcranial photobiomodulation (laser) therapy for cognitive impairment: a review of molecular mechanisms and potential application to canine cognitive dysfunction (CCD). Open Vet J 2022;12(2):256–63.
13. Brosseau L., Welch V., Wells G.A., et al., Low level laser therapy (Classes I, II and III) for treating rheumatoid arthritis, Cochrane Database Syst Rev, 4, 2005, CD002049, Available at: https://pubmed.ncbi.nlm.nih.gov/16235295/. Accessed October 30, 2022.
14. Clarkson J.E., Worthington H.V., Furness S., et al., Interventions for treating oral mucositis for patients with cancer receiving treatment, Cochrane Database Syst Rev, 8, 2010, CD001973, Available at: https://pubmed.ncbi.nlm.nih.gov/20687070/. Accessed October 30, 2022.

15. Fleming P.S., Strydom H., Katsaros C., et al., Non-pharmacological interventions for alleviating pain during orthodontic treatment, *Cochrane Database Syst Rev*, 12, 2016, CD010263, Available at: https://pubmed.ncbi.nlm.nih.gov/28009052/. Accessed October 30, 2022.
16. Page M.J., Green S., Mrocki M.A., et al., Electrotherapy modalities for rotator cuff disease, *Cochrane Database Syst Rev*, 6, 2016, CD012225, Available at: https://pubmed.ncbi.nlm.nih.gov/27283591/. Accessed October 30, 2022.
17. Page M.J., Green S., Kramer S., et al., Electrotherapy modalities for adhesive capsulitis (frozen shoulder), *Cochrane Database Syst Rev*, 10, 2014, CD011324, Available at: https://www.cochranelibrary.com/cdsr/doi/10.1002/14651858.CD011324/full. Accessed October 30, 2022.
18. Rankin I.A., Sargeant H., Rehman H., et al., Low-level laser therapy for carpal tunnel syndrome, *Cochrane Database Syst Rev*, 8, 2017, CD012765. Available at: https://www.ncbi.nlm.nih.gov/pmc/articles/PMC6483673/. Accessed October 30, 2022.
19. Yousefi-Nooraie R., Schonstein E., Heidari K., et al., Low level laser therapy for nonspecific low-back pain, *Cochrane Database Syst Rev*, 2, 2008, CD005107, Available at: https://pubmed.ncbi.nlm.nih.gov/18425909/. Accessed October 30, 2022.
20. Rosso M, Buchaim D, Kawano N, et al. Photobiomodulation therapy (PBMT) in peripheral nerve regeneration: a systematic review. Bioengineering 2018;5(2):44.
21. Huang Z, Ma J, Chen J, et al. The effectiveness of low-level laser therapy for nonspecific chronic low back pain: a systematic review and meta-analysis. Arthritis Res Ther 2015;17(1):360.
22. Huang Z, Chen J, Ma J, et al. Effectiveness of low-level laser therapy in patients with knee osteoarthritis: a systematic review and meta-analysis. Osteoarthritis Cartilage 2015;23:A384.
23. Tumilty S, Munn J, McDonough S, et al. Low level laser treatment of tendinopathy: a systematic review with meta-analysis. Photomed Laser Surg 2010;28(1):3–16.
24. Clijsen R, Brunner A, Barbero M, et al. Effects of low-level laser therapy on pain in patients with musculoskeletal disorders: a systematic review and meta-analysis. Eur J Phys Rehabil Med 2017;53(4):603–10.
25. Hochman-Elam LN, Heidel RE, Shmalberg JW. Effects of laser power, wavelength, coat length, and coat color on tissue penetration using photobiomodulation in healthy dogs. Can J Vet Res 2020;84(2):131–7.
26. Piao D, Sypniewski LA, Dugat D, et al. Transcutaneous transmission of photobiomodulation light to the spinal canal of dog as measured from cadaver dogs using a multi-channel intra-spinal probe. Lasers Med Sci 2019;34(8):1645–54.
27. Anderson KL, Zulch H, O'Neill DG, et al. Risk factors for canine osteoarthritis and its predisposing arthropathies: a systematic review. Front Vet Sci 2020;(7):220. https://doi.org/10.3389/fvets.2020.00220.
28. Enomoto M, Lascelles BDX, Gruen ME. Development of a checklist for the detection of degenerative joint disease-associated pain in cats. J Feline Med Surg 2020;22(12):1137–47.
29. Barger BK, Bisges AM, Fox DB, et al. Low-level laser therapy for osteoarthritis treatment in dogs at missouri veterinary practices. J Am Anim Hosp Assoc 2020;56(3):139–45.
30. Alves JC, Santos A, Jorge P, et al. A randomized double-blinded controlled trial on the effects of photobiomodulation therapy in dogs with osteoarthritis. Am J Vet Res 2022;83(8).

31. de Oliveira Reusing MS, do Amaral CH, Zanettin KA, et al. Effects of hydrotherapy and low-level laser therapy in canine hip dysplasia: A randomized, prospective, blinded clinical study. Rev Veterinaire Clin 2021;56(4):177–84.

32. Looney AL, Huntingford JL, Blaeser LL, et al. A randomized blind placebo-controlled trial investigating the effects of photobiomodulation therapy (PBMT) on canine elbow osteoarthritis. Can Vet J 2018;59(9):959–66.

33. Barale L, Monticelli P, Raviola M, et al. Preliminary clinical experience of low-level laser therapy for the treatment of canine osteoarthritis-associated pain: A retrospective investigation on 17 dogs. Open Vet J 2020;10(1):116–9.

34. Alvarez LX, Repac JA, Kirkby Shaw K, et al. Systematic review of postoperative rehabilitation interventions after cranial cruciate ligament surgery in dogs. Vet Surg 2022;51(2):233–43.

35. Bayat M, Virdi A, Jalalifirouzkouhi R, et al. Comparison of effects of LLLT and LIPUS on fracture healing in animal models and patients: a systematic review. Prog Biophys Mol Biol 2018;132:3–22.

36. Kennedy KC, Martinez SA, Martinez SE, et al. Effects of low-level laser therapy on bone healing and signs of pain in dogs following tibial plateau leveling osteotomy. Am J Vet Res 2018;79(8):893–904.

37. Renwick SM, Renwick AI, Brodbelt DC, et al. Influence of class IV laser therapy on the outcomes of tibial plateau leveling osteotomy in dogs. Vet Surg 2018;47(4):507–15.

38. Rogatko CP, Baltzer WI, Tennant R. Preoperative low level laser therapy in dogs undergoing tibial plateau levelling osteotomy: A blinded, prospective, randomized clinical trial. Vet Comp Orthop Traumatol 2017;30(1):46–53.

39. Draper WE, Schubert TA, Clemmons RM, et al. Low-level laser therapy reduces time to ambulation in dogs after hemilaminectomy: a preliminary study. J Small Anim Pract 2013;54(1):57.

40. Bennaim M, Porato M, Jarleton A, et al. Preliminary evaluation of the effects of photobiomodulation therapy and physical rehabilitation on early postoperative recovery of dogs undergoing hemilaminectomy for treatment of thoracolumbar intervertebral disk disease. Am J Vet Res 2017;78(2):195–206.

41. Bruno E, Canal S, Antonucci M, et al. Perilesional photobiomodulation therapy and physical rehabilitation in post-operative recovery of dogs surgically treated for thoracolumbar disk extrusion. BMC Vet Res 2020;16(1):120.

42. Miller LA, Gross TD, De Taboada L. Retrospective observational study and analysis of two different photobiomodulation therapy protocols combined with rehabilitation therapy as therapeutic interventions for canine degenerative myelopathy. Photobiomodulation Photomed Laser Surg 2020;38(4):195–205.

43. Hoisang S, Kampa N, Seesupa S, Jitpean S. Assessment of wound area reduction on chronic wounds in dogs with photobiomodulation therapy: a randomized controlled clinical trial. Vet World 2021;14(8):2251–9.

44. Wardlaw JL, Gazzola KM, Wagoner A, et al. Laser therapy for incision healing in 9 dogs. Front Vet Sci 2018;5:349.

45. Rico-Holgado S, Ortiz-Díez G, Martín-Espada MC, Fernández-Pérez C, Baquero-Artigao MR, Suárez-Redondo M. Effect of low-level laser therapy on bacterial counts of contaminated traumatic wounds in dogs. J Lasers Med Sci 2021;12(1):e78.

46. Olivieri L, Cavina D, Radicchi G, Miragliotta V, Abramo F. Efficacy of low-level laser therapy on hair regrowth in dogs with noninflammatory alopecia: a pilot study. Vet Dermatol 2015;26(1):35-e11.

47. Schnedeker AH, Cole LK, Diaz SF, et al. Is low-level laser therapy useful as an adjunctive treatment for canine acral lick dermatitis? A randomized, double-blinded, sham-controlled study. Vet Dermatol 2021;32(2):148-e35.

48. Stich AN, Rosenkrantz WS, Griffin CE. Clinical efficacy of low-level laser therapy on localized canine atopic dermatitis severity score and localized pruritic visual analog score in pedal pruritus due to canine atopic dermatitis. Vet Dermatol 2014;25(5):464-e74.

49. Alves JC, Jorge P, Santos A. The effect of photobiomodulation therapy on the management of chronic idiopathic large-bowel diarrhea in dogs. Lasers Med Sci 2022;37(3):2045-51.

Regenerative Medicine and Rehabilitation Therapy in the Canine

Brittany Jean Carr, DVM, CCRT, DACVSMR*

KEYWORDS

- Physical rehabilitation • Rehabilitation therapy • Regenerative medicine
- Stem cell therapy • Platelet-rich plasma • Low level laser therapy
- Therapeutic exercise • Therapeutic ultrasound

KEY POINTS

- The rehabilitation therapist must understand how musculoskeletal tissues heal, how regenerative medicine therapies affect healing, and how this relates to the patient and therapeutic interventions.
- Both subjective and objective outcome measures should be used to assess the patient and monitor their progress through a rehabilitation therapy program so that adjustments can be made as needed.
- Although initial studies suggest regenerative medicine and rehabilitation therapy modalities may work synergistically to enhance tissue healing, additional study is required to fully define optional rehabilitation therapy protocols after regenerative medicine therapy in the canine.

INTRODUCTION

Regenerative medicine is commonly performed in the human, equine, and canine to help manage various musculoskeletal conditions. In the canine, regenerative medicine is frequently used to treat osteoarthritis and soft tissue injuries. The two most commonly reached for forms of regenerative medicine in the canine are platelet-rich plasma (PRP) and stem cell therapy.

Platelet-Rich Plasma in the Canine

PRP is a biological product containing the plasma fraction of autologous blood with a concentration of platelets and the associated growth factors and cytokines that is higher than baseline.[1,2] The associated growth factors and cytokines that have been correlated to tissue healing include platelet-derived growth factor (PDGF),

The Veterinary Sports Medicine and Rehabilitation Center
* Corresponding author. 4104 Liberty Highway, Anderson, SC 29621.
E-mail address: dr.brittcarrbenson@gmail.com

Vet Clin Small Anim 53 (2023) 801–827
https://doi.org/10.1016/j.cvsm.2023.02.011
0195-5616/23/© 2023 Elsevier Inc. All rights reserved.

transforming growth factor-α (TGF-α), transforming growth factor-β (TGF-β), vascular endothelial growth factor (VEGF), basic fibroblastic growth factor, epidermal growth factor, connective tissue growth factor, insulin-like growth factor (IGF), hepatocyte growth factor (HGF), and keratinocyte growth factor (**Table 1**).[3] These various growth factors and cytokines have been shown to work individually and/or synergistically to promote cell recruitment, cell migration, cell proliferation, angiogenesis, and osteogenesis.[1–5] In addition, PRP has also been shown to recruit, stimulate, and provide a scaffold for stem cells.[6–10] Thus, PRP has been used to manage numerous conditions including wound healing, osteoarthritis, and soft tissue injury in canines.[11–29]

Stem Cell Therapy in the Canine

In the canine, most research has focused on adult stem cells, specifically mesenchymal stem cells (MSCs) that are derived from either the bone marrow or adipose

Table 1
Platelet-rich plasma-based growth factors and cytokines

Growth Factors and Cytokines	Function
Platelet-derived growth factor (PDGF)	Mitogenic for mesenchymal cells and osteoblasts. Stimulates chemotaxis and mitogenesis in fibroblast, glial cells, and smooth muscle cells. Regulates collagenase secretion and collagen synthesis. Stimulates macrophage and neutrophil chemotaxis.
Transforming growth factor-α (TGF-α), Transforming growth factor-β (TGF-β)	Stimulates undifferentiated mesenchymal cell proliferation. Regulates endothelial, fibroblastic, and osteoblastic mitogenesis. Regulates collagen synthesis and collagenase secretion. Regulates mitogenic effects of other growth factors. Stimulates endothelial chemotaxis and angiogenesis. Inhibits macrophage and lymphocyte proliferation.
Vascular endothelial growth factor (VEGF)	Stimulates angiogenesis and mitogenesis for endothelial cells.
Basic fibroblastic growth factor (bFGF)	Promotes growth and differentiation of chondrocytes and osteoblasts. Mitogenic for mesenchymal cells, chondrocytes, and osteoblasts.
Epidermal growth factor (EGF)	Proliferation of keratinocytes and fibroblasts. Stimulates mitogenesis for endothelial cells.
Connective tissue growth factor (CTGF)	Stimulates angiogenesis, cartilage regeneration, fibrosis, and platelet adhesion.
Insulin-like growth factor (IGF)	Chemotactic for fibroblasts and promotes protein synthesis. Augments proliferation and differentiation of osteoblasts.
Hepatocyte growth factor (HGF)	Stimulates epithelial repair and neovascularization during wound healing.
Keratinocyte growth factor (KGF)	Regulates epithelial migration and proliferation.

tissue and have the ability to differentiate into multiple cell lines such as osteoblasts, chondrocytes, and tenocytes.[30,31] Furthermore, MSCs are of great importance because of their paracrine effects through secreting growth factors and cytokines that play important roles in tissue healing, such as VEGF, TGF-β, and interleukins (IL-1β, IL-6, and IL-8).[31,32] In addition, MSCs have immunoregulatory effects by repressing T-cell proliferation, dendritic cell maturation, B-cell activation, and cytotoxic activation of resting Natural Killer (NK) cells.[31,33–38]

To date, no evidence supports superiority of one source of MSCs over the other in terms of viability or efficacy of the derived stem cells. Once the sample is obtained, it is processed and prepared for injection. Both bone marrow-derived stem cells and adipose-derived stem cells can be processed onsite or shipped to a university or private company for processing, culturing, and banking for future use. In addition, because recent studies have shown that PRP recruits and stimulates stem cells, PRP is often combined with stem cells before injection to both activate and act as a scaffold for the stem cells.[39–45] Numerous recent studies have demonstrated the efficacy of stem cell therapy for canine osteoarthritis as well as soft tissue injury.[21,46–62]

Administration of Regenerative Medicine

Injection of regenerative medicine is a minimally invasive procedure that typically can be performed on an outpatient basis. Sedation or general anesthesia is often recommended. Intra-articular injections may be performed with or without advanced imaging (digital radiology, fluoroscopy) for guidance.[63,64] For soft tissue injuries, ultrasonography guidance ensures the accuracy of the injection as both PRP and stem cells are most effective when administered directly into the site of injury.[63,64]

Initial Recommendations Following Regenerative Medicine Therapy

Following regenerative medicine therapy, exercise restriction is typically recommended for a minimum of 14 days, which means that patients should not participate in running, jumping, or playing roughly. However, this recommendation may change based on the condition that the patient is being treated for. Patients are often prescribed medications for discomfort as needed as it is not uncommon for there to be mild discomfort associated with treatment for the first 24 to 72 hours. Medications that are initially avoided following regenerative medicine therapy include glucocorticoids, nonsteroidal anti-inflammatory drugs, and antiplatelet therapies.[3] Finally, owners are advised to monitor for signs of complication, such as infection or sterile inflammatory response.[63,65,66]

PRINCIPLES OF DEVELOPING AND IMPLEMENTING A REHABILITATION THERAPY PLAN

Rehabilitation therapy is often implemented in the treatment and management of musculoskeletal conditions in the canine. Regardless of the condition being treated or the treatment methodologies used, it is imperative to adhere to basic principles of rehabilitation therapy; regenerative medicine cases are no exception to this.

First, the rehabilitation therapist must understand that musculoskeletal tissues follow a predictable pattern of healing with distinct phases.[67] Rehabilitation therapists must thoroughly understand these phases as they relate to the patient and therapeutic interventions.[68] Furthermore, in patients who have received regenerative medicine therapy, it is equally important to understand how regenerative medicine affects tissue healing for the condition being treated.[31,63,69,70]

Next, at the initial evaluation, it is important for the rehabilitation therapist to establish a baseline database of both subjective and objective outcome measures that are relevant to the condition being treated. Subjective outcome measures may include validated client-specific outcome measure surveys and subjective gait analysis.[71–82] Objective outcome measures may include muscle girth, kinetic or kinematic gait analysis, weight-bearing at stance, and goniometry.[71,72,83–86] Based on the initial assessment, an individualized treatment plan with specific, quantifiable, and appropriate goals should be developed for each patient. In addition, a patient's progress should be monitored with both subjective and objective outcome measures. Adjustments to the rehabilitation therapy program should be made as needed.

Finally, as with any rehabilitation therapy program, client education is imperative for a successful outcome. The client is the main caregiver for the patient. Thus, it is important for the client to have a comprehensive understanding of the rehabilitation therapy plan so that they are empowered as an integral care team member. It is also important for the practitioner to communicate with the client on the recommendations and expectations so that they adhere to the home care recommendations and have a general understanding of what may lie ahead for the patient.

REGENERATIVE MEDICINE AND REHABILITATION THERAPY

Rehabilitation therapy is the targeted application of mechanical, thermal, acoustic, electrical, and/or light stimuli to enhance intrinsic tissue healing potential.[87,88] The application of rehabilitation therapy modalities is based on the clinical evidence that stimuli at a tissue or organismal level improve functional outcomes following injury or disease.[89] In human medicine, the concept of regenerative rehabilitation has been introduced as the optimized application of rehabilitation science to promote regenerative therapies.[88,90] Regenerative rehabilitation has been specifically defined as the application of rehabilitation protocols and principles together with regenerative medicine therapeutics toward the goal of optimizing functional recovery through tissue regeneration, remodeling, or repair.[89] Regenerative rehabilitation is a new area of study and much work remains to be done; however, initial studies have shown that regenerative medicine and rehabilitation therapy may work safely and synergistically to enhance tissue healing.[88–90] The goal of this discussion is to highlight relevant studies on the effects of rehabilitation therapy on regenerative medicine.

Therapeutic Exercise

The goals of therapeutic exercise are to increase muscle strength, improve flexibility, improve proprioception, reduce inflammation, reduce pain, and improve function.[68,91] Multiple studies have demonstrated the important and beneficial role of low-grade mechanical strain on tissue healing.[92] Therapeutic exercise is thus an integral component of any rehabilitation therapy program.

Therapeutic exercise is thought to have application to regenerative medicine as cells and tissues respond to mechanical stimuli.[89] Extrinsic mechanical cues are transmitted by cytoskeletal structures that communicate with cytosolic messengers and/or the nucleus to regulate gene expression and cellular behavior.[89] It has been shown in recent in vitro studies that dynamic mechanical cues are potent drivers of stem cell response and play critical roles in morphogenesis, gene expression, and collagen production.[93–97] Recent studies have also demonstrated synergy between therapeutic exercise and regenerative medicine. Multiple animal tendinopathy studies have shown that mechanical loading is regenerative to tendons and works synergistically with PRP for tendon healing.[3,98,99] Therapeutic exercise has also been combined with regenerative medicine to help manage osteoarthritis. One previous study found that in dogs with osteoarthritis who were treated with plasma rich in growth factors (PRGF) and physical rehabilitation consisting of an exercise program maintained increased kinetic gait outcome measures throughout the 180-day study period, whereas dogs treated with PRGF alone had a decline in kinetic gait outcome measures after 90 days.[17] A recent case study in seven human patients with mild to moderate knee osteoarthritis treated with stromal vascular fraction (SVF) and both land- and water-based exercise had improved pain scores, quality of life scores, and functional performance measures of mobility.[100] Although optimal therapeutic exercise programs have yet to be defined, from the initial research, gentle passive range of motion (PROM) and isometric exercises within patient comfort are generally considered to be safe and possibly beneficial.

Low-Level Laser Therapy

Low-level laser therapy (LLLT) or photobiomodulation therapy is the use of red/near-infrared light to stimulate tissue healing, reduce inflammation, and reduce pain. Cellular targets absorb specific wavelengths of light, which initiates intracellular processes to cause physiologic and biological effects, such as increasing adenosine triphosphate (ATP) production, increasing collagen synthesis, increasing cellular proliferation, increasing myofibroblast activity, increasing angiogenesis, increasing osteoblast activity, increasing local endorphin release, and altering pain threshold.[87,101,102] With its multitude of physiologic and biological effects, LLLT is commonly used in veterinary rehabilitation to modulate tissue function as it is noninvasive, painless, and easily administered. Recently, photoactivation (PAC) of both PRP and MSCs has been an increasing area of study. To date, most studies assessing the effects of laser therapy and regenerative medicine have been performed using a Class IIIb laser (average radiant power <500 mW) (**Table 2**).[103]

PAC of platelets has been shown to support optimal growth factor and cytokine concentrations.[104–107] One recent study showed that PRP was successfully activated with polychromatic light (PAC, wavelength 600–1200 nm) for 10 minutes and realized activation-dependent sustained growth factor release during 28 days.[104] Thus, this study concluded that PAC has a great potential of activation of PRP and enables sustained growth factor release from PRP.[104] Recent studies have assessed using photoactivated PRP for knee osteoarthritis and found it to be safe and efficacious.[105,106,108] In addition, recent studies also found that using laser therapy and PRP or photoactivated PRP in animals with Achilles tendon injury reduced the oxidative stress on tendon and modulated collagen production at injury site.[109,110]

PAC of MSCs has also been a new area of study. It is well documented in the literature that LLLT can increase MSC differentiation, proliferation, and survival.[111–122] In addition, LLLT combined with stem cell therapy has been shown to accelerate bone healing by stimulating angiogenesis and osteogenesis.[122–126] LLLT has also been combined with MSCs to support tendon healing by stimulating tendogenic induction, increasing fibroblast survival, improving tendon reorganization.[115,116,127]

A broad range of LLLT protocols and dosing schedules were used in these studies. Most of these studies indicate that Class IIIb LLLT is safe to use in patients treated with regenerative medicine. However, although from these studies it can be concluded that LLLT positively influences regenerative medicine therapies, further study is needed to establish optimal laser therapy protocols.

Table 2
Relevant studies pertaining to low level laser therapy and regenerative medicine

Study	Study Type	Animal Model	Regenerative Medicine Product Used	Laser Power	Laser Wavelength	Laser Fluency	Laser Frequency	Conclusions
Fornaini et al, 2017	Case report	Human (jaw osteonecrosis)	PRP gel	1 W	808 nm	not stated	2x weekly for 2 wk	Safety confirmed
Patterson et al, 2016	Double-blinded, randomized controlled clinical trial	Human (knee osteoarthritis)	PA-PRP	0.005–0.100 W	480–670 nm	2.4 J/cm²	Once	Safety confirmed
Goncalves et al, 2021	In vivo	Rat (stifle osteoarthritis)	PA-PRP (8 × 10⁵ platelets)	0.025 W	808 nm	20 J/cm²	Once	All treated groups did best, PRP + PBM better on catalase activity
Freitag et al,[105] 2013	Case report	Human (knee osteoarthritis)	PA-PRP	0.005–0.100 W	480–670 nm	2.4 J/cm²	Once	Safety confirmed
Ozaki et al,[109] 2016	In vivo	Rat (gastrocnemius injury)	PRP (4999 × 10³ platelets/μL)	0.025 W	637 nm	31.85 J/cm²	Daily for 7 d	LLLT and PRP reduced oxidative stress on tendon and modulated collagen production at injury site
Alzyoud et al,[110] 2019	In vivo	Sheep (gastrocnemius injury)	PRP (5% platelet increase)	0.150–1.2 W	625 nm and 850 nm	4 J/cm²	Once	LLLT enhances cell migration and proliferation
Cavalcanti et al,[112] 2015	In vitro	Canine	BMSC	0.05 W	660 nm	1–12 J/cm²	Once	6–12 J/cm² increased canine BMSC viability and proliferation

Elbaz-Greener et al,[120] 2017	Double-blinded, randomized controlled clinical trial	Human (acute myocardial infarction)	BMSC	0.9 W	808 nm	1 J/cm²	Once	LLLT is a safe and feasible adjunctive treatment
Gutierrez et al, 2021	In vitro	Human	APSC	100 W	650 and 880 nm	3–8 J/cm²	Once	LLLT promotes proliferation and differentiation best at 6 J/m² and 650 nm
Li et al, 2022	In vitro	Rat	TDSC	2 W	532 nm	15 J/cm²	Once	A 532 nm laser with 15 J/cm regulated the process of TDSC proliferation and upregulated tenogenic differentiation.
Min et al, 2015	In vitro/ in vivo	Rat	Human ADSC	0.835 W	830 nm	0.05 J/cm²	Daily for 2–3 d	LLLT enhanced the proliferation and viability of ADSCs. The ADSCs enhanced by LLLT could be safely applied in various clinical fields.
Peat et al,[119] 2018	In vitro	Equine	BMSC	13.0 W	1064 nm	9.77 J/cm²	Once	24 h after LLLT MSCs demonstrated significant expression of IL-10 and VEGF

(continued on next page)

Table 2
(continued)

Study	Study Type	Animal Model	Regenerative Medicine Product Used	Laser Power	Laser Wavelength	Laser Fluency	Laser Frequency	Conclusions
Yin et al,[121] 2017	In vitro	Human	BMSC	0.003–0.0045 W	660 nm	not stated	Once	LLLT increases cell migration by increasing the levels of FAK that regulates cell adhesion and migration signals in cells. Cell proliferation and viability of MSCs was also increased. Growth factors (HGF and PDGF) were also elevated.
Bai et al,[124] 2021	In vitro/ in vivo	Mouse (bone healing)	Human BMSC	0.1 W	808 nm	4.5 J/cm^2	Once	LLLT increased osteogenic differentiation and bone vascularization.
Agari et al, 2020	In vivo	Rat (bone healing)	Human ADSC	0.001–75 W	890 nm	0.972 J/cm^2	3 sessions per week for 4 or 8 wk	LLLT and ADSC accelerated bone healing of bone defect in rat model.
Fekrazad et al,[125] 2019	In vitro/in vivo	Rabbit (bone healing)	BMSC	0.030–0.2 W	660 nm and 810 nm	4 J/cm^2	Once	810 and 485 nm increased cartilage differentiation; 660 and 810 nm stimulated osteogenesis

Santinoni et al,[122] 2020	In vitro/in vivo	Rat (bone healing)	BMSC	0.035 W	660 nm	4.9 J/cm² per point (39.2 J/cm² total)	Once	LLLT-enhanced angiogenesis, cell proliferation, osteoblast differentiation, and mineralization via higher VEGF, PCNA, BMP-2, OPN, and OCN expression.
Wang et al,[126] 2018	In vivo	Rat (bone healing)	Human ADSC	0.07 W	660 nm	4 J/cm²	Once	LLLT and ADSC improved fracture repair in bone defects and strong signals of vWF expression
Gomiero et al,[127] 2016	In vitro	Equine (tendon healing)	PB-MSC	25 W	660 nm and 905 nm	5 J/cm²	Once daily for 5 d	LLLT increased Tenascin C levels
Hendudari et al,[115] 2016	In vitro	Human (tendon healing)	BMSC	0.00185 W/cm²	632.8 nm	0.5, 1, and 2 J/cm²	Once	LLLT improved viability and survival of fibroblasts
Lucke et al,[116] 2018	In vitro/in vivo	Rat (tendon healing)	ADPC	0.040 W	808 nm	50 J/cm²	Once	LLLT and ADSC group had improved collaged reorganization

Abbreviations: BMP-2, bone morphogenic protein-2; BMSC, bone marrow derived stem cell; OCN, osteocalcin; OPN, osteopontin; PBM, photobiomodulation; PCNA, proliferating cell nuclear antigen; TDSC, tendon derived stem cells; vWF, von Willebrand factor.

Therapeutic Ultrasound

Therapeutic ultrasound (TUS) is the use of either continuous or pulsed mechanical acoustic waves to induce regenerative and anti-inflammatory effects on tissues. Low-intensity ultrasound has been used in veterinary rehabilitation to induce biological effects on tissues, such as accelerating tissue healing, reducing swelling, improving bone repair, reducing muscle spasm, improving tissue extensibility, and reducing pain.[87,128]

There is little available in the literature in regard to the effect of TUS on PRP. In one recent preclinical study, TUS and PRP were combined to treat stifle osteoarthritis in a guinea pig model and concluded that the group treated with TUS and PRP had improved joint lubrication as the friction coefficients reached near normal values and showed no significant difference with the normal control group.[129] Another preclinical study assessed the effect of TUS and PRP on peripheral nerve regeneration in rabbits and found that the group treated with TUS and PRP had better early axonal regeneration and displayed the earliest positive compound muscle action potential, a significant increase in myelinated nerve fiber density and diameter and myelin sheath thickness, and the best improvement of tissue stiffness and perfusion parameters on diagnostic ultrasound.[130] Unfortunately, no clinical studies have been performed evaluating TUS and PRP. Further study is necessary to elucidate the effect of TUS on PRP.

Multiple in vitro studies have assessed the effect of TUS on stem cells and demonstrated that low intensity pulsed ultrasound (LIPUS) can increase osteogenic differentiation, chondrogenic differentiation, and cell migration.[128,131–139] One recent review concluded that TUS significantly increases the level of stem cell differentiation, mainly in cells derived from bone marrow MSCs.[131] However, this review also discussed the need for further studies to analyze the effect of TUS on cells derived from other sources, particularly adipose-derived MSCs.[131] In addition, this review also cited a lack of reporting on standard TUS parameters in the literature and the need for more experiments comparing the protocols for standardization of TUS parameters to establish the best protocol.[131] Future studies are needed to clarify these discrepancies, establish efficacy, and optimal treatment protocols.

Extracorporeal Shockwave Therapy

Extracorporeal shockwave therapy (ESWT) is high-intensity acoustic waves to deliver mechanical forces to the tissue to reduce inflammatory reactions, enhance angiogenesis, suppress oxidative stress and apoptosis, and regulate stromal cell derived factor-1 (SDF-1).[87,140,141] ESWT has been used in veterinary rehabilitation therapy to treat both soft tissue injuries and osteoarthritis.[141–148]

Recently, there has been great interest in combining ESWT with regenerative medicine. One recent in vitro study demonstrated that ESWT increased growth factor concentrations in equine PRP.[149] Another experimental study in sheep with Achilles tendon injury demonstrated that the group treated with PRP and radial pressure wave therapy had increased neovascularization.[150] However, in this same study, the group treated with adipose-derived stem cells and radial pressure wave therapy had superior outcome with the highest number of thick collagen fibers and lower cellularity.[150] Unfortunately, few clinical studies evaluating ESWT and PRP have been completed. Two randomized controlled clinical trials in humans did not show an additional benefit to combining PRP and ESWT for the management of knee osteoarthritis or carpal tunnel syndrome.[151,152]

Experimental studies have also assessed the effect of ESWT on stem cells (**Table 3**). Multiple in vitro studies have demonstrated that ESWT increases rat,

Table 3
Relevant studies pertaining to the effects of ESWT on stem cells

Study	Study Type	Animal Model	Regenerative Medicine Product Used	ESWT Treatment Protocol	ESWT Treatment Frequency	Conclusions
Alshiri et al, 2020	In vitro	Goat (bone healing)	BMSC	500 shocks, 0.4 mJ/mm^2	Once	Significantly more proliferation (twofold) and osteogenic differentiation. No effect on cell motility. Further investigation for boney defects
Yin et al,[111] 2018	In vivo	Rat (soft tissue injury)	ADSC	120 impulses at 0.12 mJ/mm^2 at 3 h/24 h/72 h	Three treatments, one at 3 h/24 h/72 h post-injury	Serum levels of myoglobin and CPK lowest in ESWT + ADSC, Significantly more muscle creation in ESWT + ADSC, oxidative stress, inflammation, fibrosis and apoptosis/DNA damage were least in ESWT + ADSC
Hsu et al,[158] 2020	In vivo	Rat (stifle osteoarthritis)	ADSC vs WJMSC	1 wk post-ACL transection and meniscectomy; 800 impulses 0.25 mJ/mm^2	Once performed 30 min after SC injection	ESWT + ADSC had synergistic effect for treatment of early knee OA
Rinella et al,[155] 2018	In vitro	Human (tendon healing)	ADSC	1000 shocks, energy flux density = 0.32 mJ/mm^2; peak positive pressure 90 Mpa	Once	Combination improved differentiation toward tenoblast like cells: ESWT + ADSC had improved expression of tendon transcription factors scleraxis and eyes absent 2, and of the ECM proteins fibronectin, collagen I, and tenomodulin; Cells had acquired elongated and spindle shaped fibroblastic

(continued on next page)

Table 3
(continued)

Study	Study Type	Animal Model	Regenerative Medicine Product Used	ESWT Treatment Protocol	ESWT Treatment Frequency	Conclusions
						morphology; Collagen fibers present; combined treatment induced the expression of alpha 2, alpha 6, and beta 1 integrin subunits
Cheng et al,[164] 2019	In vivo	Rat (stifle osteoarthritis)	WJMSC	800 impulses 0.25 mJ/mm^2	Once; 30 min after WJMSC injection	ESWT + WJMSC had significantly improved early knee OA based on pathologic findings, micro-CT, and immunohistochemistry stain: increased bone volume, increased trabecular thickness, reduced synovitis
Zhang et al,[154] 2017	In vitro	Mouse	NSC	500 impulses, 2 Hz	Once	ESWT + NSC significantly improved proliferation and differentiation
Zhang et al,[153] 2018	In vitro	Rabbit (cartilage healing)	Human BMSC	Radial shockwave, 1000 impulses, 5 Hz, 200 s	Once	ESWT + MSC promoted proliferation and self-renewal of MSCs in vitro and safely accelerated the cartilage repair process in vivo
Tan et al, 2017	In vitro	Human (cartilage healing)	Human BMSC	Number of shocks varied, energy flux density = 0.18 mJ/mm^2	Once for at least 10 min	ESWT + MSC inhibits chondrogenic differentiation

Study						Findings
Suhr et al,[163] 2013	In vitro	Human	Human BMSC	1000 shocks, 4 Hz, 0.2–0.3 mJ/mm²	Once	ESWT significantly increased hBMSCs' growth rate, proliferation, migration, and cell tracking and wound healing, as well as to reduce the rate of apoptosis activation. The increase in hBMSC migration behavior was found to be mediated by active remodeling of the actin cytoskeleton as indicated by increased directed stress fiber formations. hBMSCs maintain their differentiation potentials after ESWT. 0.2 mJ/mm² was the most effective application
Raabe et al,[160] 2013	In vitro	Equine	ADSC	1000–2000 shocks	3–9 pulses	ESWT increased proliferation and expression of C×43, as detected by means of qRT-PCR, histologic staining, immunocytochemistry and western blot. Cells responded to ESWT by significant activation (phosphorylation) of ERK1/2, detected in western blots. No significant differences between treatment groups.

(continued on next page)

Table 3
(continued)

Study	Study Type	Animal Model	Regenerative Medicine Product Used	ESWT Treatment Protocol	ESWT Treatment Frequency	Conclusions
Salcedo-Jimenez et al,[159] 2020	In vitro	Equine	Umbilical Cord Blood MSC	300 shocks, energy flux density = 0.1 mJ/mm², frequency of 3 Hz	Once	ESWT-treated cells had increased metabolic activity, showed positive adipogenic, osteogenic, and chondrogenic differentiation, and showed higher potential for differentiation toward the adipogenic and osteogenic cell fates. ESWT-treated cells showed similar immunomodulatory properties to none-ESWT-treated cells
Priglinger et al,[156] 2017	In vitro	Human	SVF	200 pulses, energy flux density = 0.09 mJ/mm², frequency of 3 Hz	Once	ESWT-enhanced cellular ATP and modified expression of single mesenchymal and vascular marker. SVF + ESWT had higher IGF-1 and PLGF

Abbreviations: ACL, anterior cruciate ligament; ADSC, adipose derived stem cell; CPK, creatinine phosphokinase; ECM, extracellular matrix; ERK, extracellular signal-regulated kinase; NSC, neural stem cell; OA, osteoarthritis; qRT-PCR, quantitative reverse transcription polymerase chain reaction; WJMSC, Wharton's Jelly mesenchymal stem cell.

human, and equine MSC proliferation, differentiation, and migration.[153–163] Specifically, in vitro studies have shown that ESWT treated MSCs have shown positive adipogenic, osteogenic, and chondrogenic differentiation and showed higher potential for differentiation toward adipogenic and osteogenic cell fates.[159–163] Two recent experimental studies in rats with induced knee osteoarthritis concluded that ESWT and stem cells had a synergistic effect and the rats treated with either Wharton's jelly MSCs or adipose-derived MSCs had significant improvement based on pathologic findings, micro-CT, and immunohistochemistry stain.[164] However, to date, clinical trials have not been performed in humans or animals.

Although the initial reports in the literature are encouraging, significant additional study is required to determine the preferred treatment protocol and efficacy of ESWT and regenerative medicine to treat osteoarthritis and soft tissue injury.

REGENERATIVE MEDICINE AND MULTIMODAL REHABILITATION THERAPY

Often in veterinary rehabilitation therapy, a multimodal approach is used to holistically treat the patient. The primary injury as well as compensatory or secondary conditions are commonly addressed using multiple modalities or techniques. Unfortunately, there are limited studies in patients who have received regenerative medicine and participated in multimodal rehabilitation therapy afterward.

In one recent study, dogs with supraspinatus tendinopathy were treated with adipose-derived progenitor cell (ADPC) therapy and PRP (ADPC-PRP) combination therapy.[61] Patients were then entered into a rehabilitation therapy program that consisted of once weekly manual/massage therapy, Class IIIb LLLT for the affected shoulder (5 J/cm^2) and a twice daily at home exercise program for the first 8 weeks. In addition, at 8 weeks following treatment, patients were allowed to start hydrotherapy with underwater treadmill. In this study, it was noted that 45.5% of patients had tried rehabilitation therapy before study admission and found it to be unsuccessful.[61] At 90 days post-ADPC-PRP combination therapy and rehabilitation therapy, there was a significant improvement in temporospatial gait analysis and significant improvement in diagnostic musculoskeletal ultrasound findings.[61]

In another retrospective study, 36 dogs with partial cranial cruciate ligament (CCL) injury (<25%) were treated with stem cell and PRP combination therapy.[59] Patients were then entered into a rehabilitation therapy program that consisted of once weekly manual/massage therapy, Class IIIb LLLT for the affected stifle (5 J/cm2), and a twice daily at home exercise program for the first 8 weeks. In addition, at 8 weeks following treatment, patients were allowed to start hydrotherapy with underwater treadmill. At 90 days post-stem cell-PRP combination therapy and rehabilitation therapy, of the 13 dogs that had stifle arthroscopy findings available, nine were found to have a fully intact CCL with marked neovascularization and a normal fiber pattern in all previous regions of disruption healed.[59] Of the 11 dogs that had temporospatial gait analysis findings available, all 11 dogs had a significant improvement in total pressure index percent at 90 days.[59]

Neither of these retrospective studies had a control group, so it is very difficult to determine what role the multimodal rehabilitation therapy plan played in patient outcome. However, from these studies, it can be concluded that the multimodal rehabilitation therapy plan used in these studies seems to be safe. Additional study is required to determine how rehabilitation therapy modalities affect one another, regenerative medicine therapies, and the patient.

CLINICAL APPLICATIONS OF REHABILITATION THERAPY FOLLOWING REGENERATIVE MEDICINE

Unfortunately, evidence-based protocols are far from having been established in the veterinary literature. However, when approaching a patient treated with regenerative medicine, the rehabilitation therapists should strive to do the following:

- Discussing appropriate home care, such as exercise restrictions and environmental modifications
- Addressing pain management as needed with the assistance of the overseeing veterinarian
- Objectively assessing the patient's progress over the course of the rehabilitation therapy program
- Communicating with the overseeing veterinarian to express concerns regarding the patient
- Educating the client on the patient's condition, rehabilitation therapy plan, medical recommendations, and patient progress

In addition, from the initial studies, the rehabilitation therapist should feel comfortable administering the following therapies for the first 4 to 8 weeks after regenerative medicine:

- Gentle PROM and stretching within the patient's comfort
- Isometric exercise program within the patient's comfort and ability
- Manual/massage therapy for all areas of compensatory tension or discomfort

Given the lack of literature available regarding various rehabilitation modalities, rehabilitation modalities should be used cautiously at the site of treatment. Although Class IIIb LLLT (average radiant power <500 mW) seems to be safe at the site of injury, optimal dosing parameters and efficacy have not been established. The evidence for TUS is encouraging but limited, so it is not commonly reached for clinically following regenerative medicine. Although the initial in vitro studies regarding ESWT and regenerative medicine are positive, there are limited in vivo studies. Ultimately, additional studies in the species of interest are needed to establish the effects of rehabilitation modalities on regenerative medicine and to establish evidence-based protocols.

VETERINARY REGENERATIVE REHABILITATION: CHALLENGES AND FUTURE DIRECTIONS

Further research is needed to elucidate the effect of rehabilitation therapy on regenerative medicine therapies. Although in vitro studies are essential for understanding molecular and cellular responses to biophysical signals, the application of these studies to clinical treatments is limited in that these studies do not account for functional communication and interactions between neighboring tissues and cell systems or the patient as a whole. Likewise, pathologic conditions often alter mechanotransductive cascades and cell mechanics, which are sometimes challenging to recreate in an in vitro study. Experimental in vivo studies attempt to recreate a pathologic state but still fail to recreate a true clinical scenario of tissue injury or impaired mobility. In spite of these limitations, in vitro and experimental in vivo studies are still of great value and foundational preclinical studies. These experimental studies provide a starting point for randomized controlled clinical trials in the species of interest that assess objective outcome measures, which are required to establish evidence-based protocols.

In addition, in the literature, there is a significant lack of description of the regenerative medicine products and the rehabilitation protocols used. Few studies provide a complete description of the regenerative medicine product used in the study, such as product constituents, source, cell number, route of administration, timing of administration after surgery/injury and in relation to rehabilitation, and so forth. Likewise, there is often insufficient description of the key parameters of the rehabilitation protocol, such as timing after surgery/injury, frequency, intensity, dose, duration, and so forth. All of these characteristics and parameters can play a significant role in patient outcome. It is imperative that future studies standardize nomenclature and thoroughly clarify products and protocols being used. This is of the utmost importance if evidence-based protocols are to be established.

In summary, regenerative medicine is certain to become standard of care as additional studies become available further elucidating its use and efficacy. Additional study is required to fully clarify the role of rehabilitation therapy in patients who have received regenerative medicine. In the emergence of this field of study, regenerative rehabilitation represents the interface of two disciplines serving the same goal to accelerate tissue restoration after injury and disease. This new frontier of research is needed to further define how regenerative medicine and rehabilitation interact to optimize and enhance tissue healing and patient outcome.

CLINICS CARE POINTS

- The rehabilitation therapist should have a comprehensive understanding of the pattern musculoskeletal tissues follow during healing and how this relates to the patient who has received regenerative medicine therapy.
- The rehabilitation therapist should use both subjective and objective outcome measures to assess the patient and monitor their progress and adjust the program as needed.
- Initial studies suggest that gentle passive range of motion and stretching within the patient's comfort and isometric exercises may be safe and beneficial for patients treated with regenerative medicine therapy.[3,17,89–100]
- Initial studies have shown that Class IIIb low-level laser therapy (LLLT) can be safely applied to platelet-rich plasma and mesenchymal stem cells; however, optimal LLLT protocols and clinical efficacy have not been established.[104–127]
- Additional study is required to fully define optional rehabilitation therapy protocols after regenerative medicine therapy in the canine, and it is imperative that future studies standardize nomenclature and thoroughly clarify products and protocols being used so that specific evidence-based protocols can be developed.

DISCLOSURE

The author is a consultant for Companion Animal Health.

REFERENCES

1. Alves R, Grimalt R. A review of platelet-rich plasma: history, biology, mechanism of action, and classification. Skin Appendage Disord 2018;4(1):18–24.
2. Arnoczky SP, Sheibani-Rad S. The basic science of platelet-rich plasma (PRP): what clinicians need to know. Sports Med Arthrosc Rev 2013;21(4):180–5, published correction appears in Sports Med Arthrosc. 2014;22(2):150. Shebani-Rad, Shahin [corrected to Sheibani-Rad, Shahin.

3. Everts P, Onishi K, Jayaram P, et al. Platelet-rich plasma: new performance understandings and therapeutic considerations in 2020. Int J Mol Sci 2020;21(20): 7794.

4. Hudgens JL, Sugg KB, Grekin JA, et al. Platelet-rich plasma activates proinflammatory signaling pathways and induces oxidative stress in tendon fibroblasts. Am J Sports Med 2016;44(8):1931–40.

5. Andia I, Rubio-Azpeitia E, Maffulli N. Platelet-rich plasma modulates the secretion of inflammatory/angiogenic proteins by inflamed tenocytes. Clin Orthop Relat Res 2015;473(5):1624–34.

6. Lai F, Kakudo N, Morimoto N, et al. Platelet-rich plasma enhances the proliferation of human adipose stem cells through multiple signaling pathways. Stem Cell Res Ther 2018;9(1):107.

7. Tobita M, Tajima S, Mizuno H. Adipose tissue-derived mesenchymal stem cells and platelet-rich plasma: stem cell transplantation methods that enhance stemness. Stem Cell Res Ther 2015;6:215.

8. Ricco S, Renzi S, Del Bue M, et al. Allogeneic adipose tissue-derived mesenchymal stem cells in combination with platelet rich plasma are safe and effective in the therapy of superficial digital flexor tendonitis in the horse. Int J Immunopathol Pharmacol 2013;26(1 Suppl):61–8.

9. Martinello T, Bronzini I, Perazzi A, et al. Effects of in vivo applications of peripheral blood-derived mesenchymal stromal cells (PB-MSCs) and platlet-rich plasma (PRP) on experimentally injured deep digital flexor tendons of sheep. J Orthop Res 2013;31(2):306–14.

10. Zhang J, Wang JH. Platelet-rich plasma releasate promotes differentiation of tendon stem cells into active tenocytes. Am J Sports Med 2010;38(12):2477–86.

11. Farghali HA, AbdElKader NA, Khattab MS, et al. Evaluation of subcutaneous infiltration of autologous platelet-rich plasma on skin-wound healing in dogs. Biosci Rep 2017;37(2). BSR20160503.

12. Farghali HA, AbdElKader NA, AbuBakr HO, et al. Antimicrobial action of autologous platelet-rich plasma on MRSA-infected skin wounds in dogs. Sci Rep 2019;9(1):12722.

13. Jee CH, Eom NY, Jang HM, et al. Effect of autologous platelet-rich plasma application on cutaneous wound healing in dogs. J Vet Sci 2016;17(1):79–87.

14. Iacopetti I, Patruno M, Melotti L, et al. Autologous platelet-rich plasma enhances the healing of large cutaneous wounds in dogs. Front Vet Sci 2020;7:575449.

15. Marshall W, Bockstahler B, Hulse D, et al. A review of osteoarthritis and obesity: current understanding of the relationship and benefit of obesity treatment and prevention in the dog. Vet Comp Orthop Traumatol 2009;22(5):339–45.

16. Kazemi D, Fakhrjou A. Leukocyte and platelet rich plasma (l-prp) versus leukocyte and platelet rich fibrin (l-prf) for articular cartilage repair of the knee: a comparative evaluation in an animal model. Iran Red Crescent Med J 2015; 17(10):e19594.

17. Cuervo B, Rubio M, Chicharro D, et al. Objective comparison between platelet rich plasma alone and in combination with physical therapy in dogs with osteoarthritis caused by hip dysplasia. Animals (Basel) 2020;10(2):175.

18. Catarino J, Carvalho P, Santos S, et al. Treatment of canine osteoarthritis with allogeneic platelet-rich plasma: review of five cases. Open Vet J 2020;10(2): 226–31.

19. Venator KP, Frye CW, Gamble LJ, et al. Assessment of a Single Intra-Articular Stifle Injection of Pure Platelet Rich Plasma on Symmetry Indices in Dogs with

Unilateral or Bilateral Stifle Osteoarthritis from Long-Term Medically Managed Cranial Cruciate Ligament Disease. Vet Med (Auckl) 2020;11:31–8.

20. Vilar JM, Manera ME, Santana A, et al. Effect of leukocyte-reduced platelet-rich plasma on osteoarthritis caused by cranial cruciate ligament rupture: A canine gait analysis model. PLoS One 2018;13(3):e0194752.

21. Okamoto-Okubo CE, Cassu RN, Joaquim JGF, et al. Chronic pain and gait analysis in dogs with degenerative hip joint disease treated with repeated intra-articular injections of platelet-rich plasma or allogeneic adipose-derived stem cells. J Vet Med Sci 2021;83(5):881–8.

22. Alves JC, Santos A, Jorge P, et al. A report on the use of a single intra-articular administration of autologous platelet therapy in a naturally occurring canine osteoarthritis model - a preliminary study. BMC Musculoskelet Disord 2020; 21(1):127.

23. Alves JC, Santos A, Jorge P. Platelet-rich plasma therapy in dogs with bilateral hip osteoarthritis. BMC Vet Res 2021;17(1):207.

24. Bozynski CC, Stannard JP, Smith P, et al. Acute Management of Anterior Cruciate Ligament Injuries Using Novel Canine Models. J Knee Surg 2016;29(7): 594–603.

25. Cook JL, Smith PA, Bozynski CC, et al. Multiple injections of leukoreduced platelet rich plasma reduce pain and functional impairment in a canine model of ACL and meniscal deficiency. J Orthop Res 2016;34(4):607–15.

26. Franklin SP, Franklin AL. Randomized Controlled Trial Comparing Autologous Protein Solution to Hyaluronic Acid Plus Triamcinolone for Treating Hip Osteoarthritis in Dogs. Front Vet Sci 2021;8:713768.

27. Xie X, Wu H, Zhao S, et al. The effect of platelet-rich plasma on patterns of gene expression in a dog model of anterior cruciate ligament reconstruction. J Surg Res 2013;180(1):80–8.

28. Xie X, Zhao S, Wu H, et al. Platelet-rich plasma enhances autograft revascularization and reinnervation in a dog model of anterior cruciate ligament reconstruction. J Surg Res 2013;183(1):214–22.

29. Ho LK, Baltzer WI, Nemanic S, et al. Single ultrasound-guided platelet-rich plasma injection for treatment of supraspinatus tendinopathy in dogs. Can Vet J 2015;56(8):845–9.

30. Freitag J, Bates D, Boyd R, et al. Mesenchymal stem cell therapy in the treatment of osteoarthritis: reparative pathways, safety and efficacy - a review. BMC Musculoskelet Disord 2016;17:230.

31. Kangari P, Talaei-Khozani T, Razeghian-Jahromi I, et al. Mesenchymal stem cells: amazing remedies for bone and cartilage defects. Stem Cell Res Ther 2020;11(1):492.

32. Hofer HR, Tuan RS. Secreted trophic factors of mesenchymal stem cells support neurovascular and musculoskeletal therapies. Stem Cell Res Ther 2016; 7(1):131.

33. Mea DN. Human bone marrow stromal cells suppress T-lymphocyte proliferation induced by cellular or nonspecific mitogenic stimuli. Blood 2002;99:3838–43.

34. Spaggiari GM, Capobianco A, Becchetti S, et al. Mesenchymal stem cell– natural killer cell interactions: evidence that activated NK cells are capable of killing MSCs, whereas MSCs can inhibit IL-2-induced NK-cell proliferation. Blood 2006;107:1484–90.

35. Yagi HS-GA, Parekkadan B, Kitagawa Y, et al. Mesenchymal stem cells: mechanisms of immunomodulation and homing. Cell Transpl 2010;19:667–79.

36. Sun YQDM, He J, Zeng QX, et al. Human pluripotent stem cell-derived mesenchymal stem cells prevent allergic airway inflammation in mice. Stem Cells 2012; 30:2692–9.
37. Chabannes DHM, Merieau E, Rossignol J, et al. A role for heme oxygenase-1 in the immunosuppressive effect of adult rat and human mesenchymal stem cells. Blood 2007;110:3691–4.
38. Fu QLCY, Sun SJ, Zeng QX, et al. Mesenchymal stem cells derived from human induced pluripotent stem cells modulate T-cell phenotypes in allergic rhinitis. Allergy 2012;67(10):1215–22.
39. Carvalho AM, Badial PR, Alvarez LE, et al. Equine tendonitis therapy using mesenchymal stem cells and platelet concentrations: A randomized controlled trial. Stem Cell Res Ther 2013;22(4):85.
40. Del Bue M, Ricco S, Ramoni R, et al. Equine adipose-tissue derived mesenchymal stem cells and platelet concentrations: Their association in vitro and in vivo. Vet Res Commun 2008;32(1):S51–5.
41. Chen L, Dong SW, Liu JP, et al. Synergy of tendon stem cells and platelet-rich-plasma in tendon healing. J Orthop Res 2012;30(6):991–7.
42. Uysal CA, Tobita M, Hyakusoku H, et al. Adipose-derived stem cells enhance primary tendon repair: Biomechanical and immunohistochemical evaluation. J Plast Reconstr Aesthet Surg 2012;65(12):1712–9.
43. Manning CN, Schwartz AG, Liu W, et al. Controlled delivery of mesenchymal stem cells and growth factors using a nanofiber scaffold for tendon repair. Acta Biomater 2013;9(6):6905–14.
44. Yun JH, Han SH, Choi SH, et al. Effects of bone marrow-derived mesenchymal stem cells and platelet-rich plasma on bone regeneration for osseointegration of dental implants: Preliminary study in canine three-wall intrabony defects. J Biomed Mater Res B Appl Biomater 2014;102(5):1021–30.
45. Tobita M, Uysal CA, Guo X, et al. Periodontal tissue regeneration by combined implantation of adipose tissue-derived stem cells and platelet-rich plasma in a canine model. Cryotherapy 2013;15(12):1517–26.
46. Kiefer KM, Lin K, Fitzpatrick N, et al. Does Adipose-Derived Stromal Cell Adjuvant Therapy for Fragmented Medial Coronoid Process in Dogs Influence Outcome? A Pilot Project. Vet evid 2016;1(4). https://doi.org/10.18849/ve.v1i4.45.
47. Black LL, Gaynor J, Adams C, et al. Effect of intraarticular injection of autologous adipose-derived mesenchymal stem and regenerative cells on clinical signs of chronic osteoarthritis of the elbow joint in dogs. Vet Ther 2008;9(3): 192–200.
48. Guercio A, Di Marco P, Casella S, et al. Production of canine mesenchymal stem cells from adipose tissue and their application in dogs with chronic osteoarthritis of the humeroradial joints. Cell Biol Int 2012;36:189–94.
49. Cuervo B, Rubio M, Sopena J, et al. Hip osteoarthritis in dogs: a randomized study using mesenchymal stem cells from adipose tissue and plasma rich in growth factors. Int J Mol Sci 2014;15:13437–60.
50. Black LL, Gaynor J, Gahring D, et al. Effect of adipose-derived mesenchymal stem and regenerative cells on lameness in dogs with chronic osteoarthritis of the coxofemoral joints: a randomized, double-blinded, multicenter, controlled trial. Vet Ther 2007;8(4):272–84.
51. Vilar JM, Morales M, Santana A, et al. Controlled, blinded force platform analysis of the effect of intraarticular injection of autologous adipose-derived mesenchymal stem cells associated to PRGF-Endoret in osteoarthritic dogs. BMC Vet Res 2013;9:131.

52. Vilar JM, Batista M, Morales M, et al. Assessment of the effect of intraarticular injection of autologous adipose derived mesenchymal stem cells in osteoarthritic dogs using a double-blinded force platform analysis. BMC Vet Res 2014;10:143.

53. Yun S, Ku SK, Kwon YS. Adipose-derived mesenchymal stem cells and platelet-rich plasma synergistically ameliorate the surgical-induced osteoarthritis in Beagle dogs. J Orthopaedic Surg Res 2016;11:9.

54. Tsai SY, Huang YC, Chueh LL, et al. Intra-articular transplantation of porcine adipose-derived stem cells for the treatment of canine osteoarthritis: a pilot study. World J Transpl 2014;4(3):196–205.

55. Upchurch DA, Renberg WC, Roush JK, et al. Effects of administration of adipose-derived stromal vascular fraction and platelet-rich plasma to dogs with osteoarthritis of the hip joints. Am J Vet Res 2016;77(9):940–51.

56. Ivanovska A, Wang M, Arshaghi TE, et al. Manufacturing mesenchymal stromal cells for the treatment of osteoarthritis in canine patients: challenges and recommendations. Front Vet Sci 2022;9:897150.

57. Sanghani-Kerai A, Black C, Cheng SO, et al. Clinical outcomes following intra-articular injection of autologous adipose-derived mesenchymal stem cells for the treatment of osteoarthritis in dogs characterized by weight-bearing asymmetry. Bone Joint Res 2021;10(10):650–8.

58. Case JB, Palmer R, Valdes-Martinez A, et al. Gastrocnemius tendon strain in a dog treated with autologous mesenchymal stem cells and a custom orthosis. Vet Surg 2013;42. 355-260.

59. Canapp SO Jr, Leasure CS, Cox C, et al. Partial cranial cruciate ligament tears treated with stem cell and platelet-rich plasma combination therapy in 36 dogs: a retrospective study. Front Vet Sci 2016;3:112.

60. McDougall RA, Canapp SO, Canapp DA. Ultrasonographic findings in 41 dogs treated with bone marrow aspirate concentrate and platelet-rich plasma for a supraspinatus tendinopathy: a retrospective study. Front Vet Sci 2018;5:98.

61. Canapp SO Jr, Canapp DA, Ibrahim V, et al. The use of adipose-derived progenitor cells and platelet-rich plasma combination for the treatment of supraspinatus tendinopathy in 55 dogs: a retrospective study. Front Vet Sci 2016;3:61.

62. Xiao WF, Yang YT, Xie WQ, et al. Effects of platelet-rich plasma and bone marrow mesenchymal stem cells on meniscal repair in the white-white zone of the meniscus. Orthop Surg 2021;13(8):2423–32.

63. Carr BJ. Platelet-rich plasma as an orthobiologic: clinically relevant considerations. Vet Clin North Am Small Anim Pract 2022;52(4):977–95.

64. Malanga GA, Ibrahim V. Regenerative treatments in Sports and orthopedic medicine. Demos Medical; 2017.

65. Eymard F, Ornetti P, Maillet J, et al. Correction to: Intra-articular injections of platelet-rich plasma in symptomatic knee osteoarthritis: a consensus statement from French-speaking experts. Knee Surg Sports Traumatol Arthrosc 2021; 29(10):3211–2.

66. Eliasberg CD, Nemirov DA, Mandelbaum BR, et al. Complications following biologic therapeutic injections: a multicenter case series. Arthroscopy 2021;37(8): 2600–5.

67. Cornell K. Wound Healing. In: Tobias KM, Johnston SA, editors. Veterinary surgery: small animal. 1st ed. St. Louis, MO: Elsvier; 2012. p. 125–34.

68. Kirkby Shaw K, Alvarez L, Foster SA, et al. Fundamental principles of rehabilitation and musculoskeletal tissue healing. Vet Surg 2020;49(1):22–32.

69. Lui PP. Stem cell technology for tendon regeneration: current status, challenges, and future research directions. Stem Cells Cloning 2015;8:163–74.

70. Zeng N, Chen H, Wu Y, et al. Adipose stem cell-based treatments for wound healing. Front Cell Dev Biol 2022;9:821652.

71. Zink MC, Carr BJ, Zink MC, et al. Locomotion and athletic performance. Canine sports medicine and rehabilitation. Hoboken, NJ: John Wiley & Sons; 2018.

72. Levine D, Marcellin-Little DJ, Drum M, et al. The physical rehabilitation evaluation. Canine rehabilitation and physical therapy. Philadelphia, PA: Elsevier; 2014.

73. Brown DC, Boston RC, Coyne JC, et al. Development and psychometric testing of an instrument designed to measure chronic pain in dogs with osteoarthritis. Am J Vet Res 2007 Jun;68(6):631–7.

74. Hielm-Björkman AK, Rita H, Tulamo RM. Psychometric testing of the Helsinki chronic pain index by completion of a questionnaire in Finnish by owners of dogs with chronic signs of pain caused by osteoarthritis. Am J Vet Res 2009; 70(6):727–34.

75. Brown DC. The canine orthopedic index. Step 1: Devising the items. Vet Surg 2014;43(3):232–40.

76. Brown DC. The canine orthopedic index. Step 2: Psychometric testing. Vet Surg 2014;43(3):241–6.

77. Brown DC. The canine orthopedic Index. Step 3: Responsiveness testing. Vet Surg 2014;43(3):247–54.

78. Hercock CA, Pinchbeck G, Giejda A, et al. Validation of a client-based clinical metrology instrument for the evaluation of canine elbow osteoarthritis. J Small Anim Pract 2009;50(6):266–71.

79. Hudson JT, Slater MR, Taylor L, et al. Assessing repeatability and validity of a visual analogue scale questionnaire for use in assessing pain and lameness in dogs. Am J Vet Res 2004;65(12):1634–43.

80. Reid J, Nolan AM, Hughes JML, et al. Development of the short-form Glasgow Composite Measure Pain Scale (CMPS-SF) and derivation of an analgesic intervention score. Anim Welf 2007;16(S):97–104.

81. Lavan RP. Development and validation of a survey for quality of life assessment by owners of healthy dogs. Vet J 2013 Sep;197(3):578–82.

82. Cachon T, Frykman O, Innes JF, et al, COAST Development Group. Face validity of a proposed tool for staging canine osteoarthritis: Canine OsteoArthritis Staging Tool (COAST). Vet J 2018;235:1–8.

83. Millis D, Levine D. Canine rehabilitation and physical therapy. Elsevier Health Sciences; 2013.

84. Brown DC, Boston RC, Farrar JT. Use of an activity monitor to detect response to treatment in dogs with osteoarthritis. J Am Vet Med Assoc 2010 Jul 1;237(1): 66–70.

85. Jaegger G, Marcellin-Little DJ, Levine D. Reliability of goniometry in Labrador Retrievers. Am J Vet Res 2002 Jul;63(7):979–86.

86. Freund KA, Kieves NR, Hart JL, et al. Assessment of novel digital and smartphone goniometers for measurement of canine stifle joint angles. Am J Vet Res 2016;77(7):749–55.

87. Niebaum K, McCauley L, Medina C, et al. Rehabilitation therapy modalities. Canine sports medicine and rehabilitation. Hoboken, NJ: John Wiley & Sons; 2018.

88. Ambrosio F, Wolf SL, Delitto A, et al. The emerging relationship between regenerative medicine and physical therapeutics. Phys Ther 2010;90(12):1807–14.

89. Rando TA, Ambrosio F. Regenerative rehabilitation: applied biophysics meets stem cell therapeutics [published correction appears in cell stem cell. 2018 Apr 5;22(4):608]. Cell Stem Cell 2018;22(3):306–9.

90. Tashiro S, Nakamura M, Okano H. Regenerative rehabilitation and stem cell therapy targeting chronic spinal cord injury: a review of preclinical studies. Cells 2022;11(4):685.

91. McCauley L, Van Dyke JB, Zink MC, et al. Therapeutic exercise. Canine Sports medicine and rehabilitation. Hoboken, NJ: John Wiley & Sons; 2018.

92. Bliss S, Zink MC, Van Dyke JB. Musculoskeletal structure and physiology. Canine sports medicine and rehabilitation. Hoboken, NJ: John Wiley & Sons; 2018.

93. Heisenberg CP, Bellaïche Y. Forces in tissue morphogenesis and patterning. Cell 2013;153(5):948–62.

94. Adamo L, Naveiras O, Wenzel PL, et al. Biomechanical forces promote embryonic haematopoiesis. Nature 2009;459(7250):1131–5.

95. Wong VW, Longaker MT, Gurtner GC. Soft tissue mechanotransduction in wound healing and fibrosis. Semin Cell Dev Biol 2012;23(9):981–6.

96. Asadi S, Farzanegi P, Azarbayjani MA. Combined therapies with exercise, ozone and mesenchymal stem cells improve the expression of HIF1 and SOX9 in the cartilage tissue of rats with knee osteoarthritis. Physiol Int 2020;107(2):231–42.

97. de Freitas JS, Neves CA, Del Carlo RJ, et al. Effects of exercise training and stem cell therapy on the left ventricle of infarcted rats. Rev Port Cardiol (Engl Ed 2019;38(9):649–56.

98. Neph A, Schroeder A, Enseki KR, et al. Role of Mechanical Loading for Platelet-Rich Plasma-Treated Achilles Tendinopathy. Curr Sports Med Rep 2020;19(6): 209–16.

99. Virchenko O, Aspenberg P. How can one platelet injection after tendon injury lead to a stronger tendon after 4 weeks? Interplay between early regeneration and mechanical stimulation. Acta Orthop 2006;77(5):806–12.

100. Gibbs N, Diamond R, Sekyere EO, et al. Management of knee osteoarthritis by combined stromal vascular fraction cell therapy, platelet-rich plasma, and musculoskeletal exercises: a case series. J Pain Res 2015;8:799–806.

101. Anders JJ, Kobiela Ketz A, Wu X. Basic principles of photobiomodulation and its effects at the cellular, tissue, and system levels. In: Riegel RJ, Godbold JC, editors. Laser therapy in veterinary medicine: photobiomodulation. Ames, Iowa: Wiley Blackwell; 2017. p. 36–52.

102. Mussttaf RA, Jenkins DFL, Jha AN. Assessing the impact of low level laser therapy (LLLT) on biological systems: a review. Int J Radiat Biol 2019;95(2):120–43.

103. American National Standards Institute, Inc. American National Standard for Safe Use of Lasers. 2013. Z136.1-2014. Available at: https://webstore.ansi.org/ Standards/LIA/ANSIZ1362014?gclid=CjwKCAjw7p6aBhBiEiwA83fGulP5UkiS uONCNEUOtpsH0A93sdCpU7JwumOXZTQ8HpPvZ5a0kWxKaxoCcusQAvD_ BwE. Accessed July 1, 2022.

104. Irmak G, Demirtaş TT, Gümüşderelioğlu M. Sustained release of growth factors from photoactivated platelet rich plasma (PRP). Eur J Pharm Biopharm 2020; 148:67–76.

105. Freitag JB, Barnard A. To evaluate the effect of combining photo-activation therapy with platelet-rich plasma injections for the novel treatment of osteoarthritis. BMJ Case Rep 2013;2013. bcr2012007463.

106. Paterson KL, Nicholls M, Bennell KL, et al. Intra-articular injection of photo-activated platelet-rich plasma in patients with knee osteoarthritis: a double-

blind, randomized controlled pilot study. BMC Musculoskelet Disord 2016; 17:67.

107. Zhevago NA, Samoilova KA. Pro- and anti-inflammatory cytokine content in human peripheral blood after its transcutaneous (in vivo) and direct (in vitro) irradiation with polychromatic visible and infrared light. Photomed Laser Surg 2006; 24(2):129–39.

108. Gonçalves AB, Bovo JL, Gomes BS, et al. Photobiomodulation (λ=808nm) and Platelet-Rich Plasma (PRP) for the Treatment of Acute Rheumatoid Arthritis in Wistar Rats. J Lasers Med Sci 2021;12(e60).

109. Ozaki GA, Camargo RC, Koike TE, et al. Analysis of photobiomodulation associated or not with platelet-rich plasma on repair of muscle tissue by Raman spectroscopy. Lasers Med Sci 2016;31(9):1891–8.

110. Alzyoud JAM, Al Najjar SA, Talat S, et al. Effect of light-emitting diodes, platelet-rich plasma, and their combination on the activity of sheep tenocytes. Lasers Med Sci 2019;34(4):759–66.

111. Bayat M, Virdi A, Rezaei F, et al. Comparison of the in vitro effects of low-level laser therapy and low-intensity pulsed ultrasound therapy on bony cells and stem cells. Prog Biophys Mol Biol 2018;133:36–48.

112. Cavalcanti MF, Maria DA, de Isla N, et al. Evaluation of the proliferative effects induced by low-level laser therapy in bone marrow stem cell culture. Photomed Laser Surg 2015;33(12):610–6.

113. Ginani F, Soares DM, Barreto MP, et al. Effect of low-level laser therapy on mesenchymal stem cell proliferation: a systematic review. Lasers Med Sci 2015;30(8):2189–94.

114. Gutiérrez D, Rouabhia M, Ortiz J, et al. Low-level laser irradiation promotes proliferation and differentiation on apical papilla stem cells. J Lasers Med Sci 2021; 12:e75.

115. Hendudari F, Piryaei A, Hassani SN, et al. Combined effects of low-level laser therapy and human bone marrow mesenchymal stem cell conditioned medium on viability of human dermal fibroblasts cultured in a high-glucose medium. Lasers Med Sci 2016;31(4):749–57.

116. Lucke LD, Bortolazzo FO, Theodoro V, et al. Low-level laser and adipose-derived stem cells altered remodelling genes expression and improved collagen reorganization during tendon repair. Cell Prolif 2019;52(3):e12580.

117. Li M, Zhu Y, Pei Q, et al. The 532 nm laser treatment promotes the proliferation of tendon-derived stem cells and upregulates nr4a1 to stimulate tenogenic differentiation. Photobiomodul Photomed Laser Surg 2022;40(8):543–53.

118. Min KH, Byun JH, Heo CY, et al. Effect of low-level laser therapy on human adipose-derived stem cells: in vitro and in vivo studies. Aesthet Plast Surg 2015;39(5):778–82.

119. Peat FJ, Colbath AC, Bentsen LM, et al. In vitro effects of high-intensity laser photobiomodulation on equine bone marrow-derived mesenchymal stem cell viability and cytokine expression. Photomed Laser Surg 2018;36(2):83–91.

120. Elbaz-Greener G, Sud M, Tzuman O, et al. Adjunctive laser-stimulated stem-cells therapy to primary reperfusion in acute myocardial infarction in humans: Safety and feasibility study. J Interv Cardiol 2018;31(6):711–6.

121. Yin K, Zhu R, Wang S, et al. Low-level laser effect on proliferation, migration, and antiapoptosis of mesenchymal stem cells. Stem Cells Dev 2017;26(10):762–75.

122. Santinoni CS, Neves APC, Almeida BFM, et al. Bone marrow coagulated and low-level laser therapy accelerate bone healing by enhancing angiogenesis,

cell proliferation, osteoblast differentiation, and mineralization. J Biomed Mater Res A 2021;109(6):849–58.

123. Asgari M, Gazor R, Abdollahifar MA, et al. Combined therapy of adipose-derived stem cells and photobiomodulation on accelerated bone healing of a critical size defect in an osteoporotic rat model. Biochem Biophys Res Commun 2020;530(1):173–80.

124. Bai J, Li L, Kou N, et al. Low level laser therapy promotes bone regeneration by coupling angiogenesis and osteogenesis. Stem Cell Res Ther 2021;12(1):432.

125. Fekrazad R, Asefi S, Eslaminejad MB, et al. Photobiomodulation with single and combination laser wavelengths on bone marrow mesenchymal stem cells: proliferation and differentiation to bone or cartilage. Lasers Med Sci 2019;34(1): 115–26, published correction appears in Lasers Med Sci. 2018 Dec 19.

126. Wang YH, Wu JY, Kong SC, et al. Low power laser irradiation and human adipose-derived stem cell treatments promote bone regeneration in critical-sized calvarial defects in rats. PLoS One 2018;13(4):e0195337.

127. Gomiero C, Bertolutti G, Martinello T, et al. Tenogenic induction of equine mesenchymal stem cells by means of growth factors and low-level laser technology. Vet Res Commun 2016;40(1):39–48.

128. de Lucas B, Pérez LM, Bernal A, et al. Ultrasound therapy: experiences and perspectives for regenerative medicine. Genes (Basel) 2020;11(9):1086.

129. Tavakoli J, Torkaman G, Ravanbod R, et al. Regenerative effect of low-intensity pulsed ultrasound and platelet-rich plasma on the joint friction and biomechanical properties of cartilage: a non-traumatic osteoarthritis model in the guinea pig. Ultrasound Med Biol 2022;48(5):862–71.

130. Zhu Y, Jin Z, Fang J, et al. Platelet-rich plasma combined with low-dose ultra-short wave therapy accelerates peripheral nerve regeneration. Tissue Eng A 2020;26(3–4):178–92.

131. Amini A, Chien S, Bayat M. Impact of ultrasound therapy on stem cell differentiation - a systematic review. Curr Stem Cell Res Ther 2020;15(5):462–72.

132. Garg P, Mazur MM, Buck AC, et al. Prospective review of mesenchymal stem cells differentiation into osteoblasts. Orthop Surg 2017;9(1):13–9.

133. Lai CH, Chen SC, Chiu LH, et al. Effects of low-intensity pulsed ultrasound, dexamethasone/TGF-beta1 and/or BMP-2 on the transcriptional expression of genes in human mesenchymal stem cells: chondrogenic vs. osteogenic differentiation. Ultrasound Med Biol 2010;36(6):1022–33.

134. Ning GZ, Song WY, Xu H, et al. Bone marrow mesenchymal stem cells stimulated with low-intensity pulsed ultrasound: Better choice of transplantation treatment for spinal cord injury: Treatment for SCI by LIPUS-BMSCs transplantation. CNS Neurosci Ther 2019;25(4):496–508.

135. de Lucas B, Pérez LM, Bernal A, et al. Application of low-intensity pulsed therapeutic ultrasound on mesenchymal precursors does not affect their cell properties. PLoS One 2021;16(2):e0246261.

136. Gao Q, Walmsley AD, Cooper PR, et al. Ultrasound stimulation of different dental stem cell populations: role of mitogen-activated protein kinase signaling. J Endod 2016;42(3):425–31.

137. Xia P, Wang X, Wang Q, et al. Low-intensity pulsed ultrasound promotes autophagy-mediated migration of mesenchymal stem cells and cartilage repair. Cell Transpl 2021;30. 963689720986142.

138. Lee HJ, Choi BH, Min BH, et al. Low-intensity ultrasound stimulation enhances chondrogenic differentiation in alginate culture of mesenchymal stem cells. Artif Organs 2006;30(9):707–15.

139. Wang X, Lin Q, Zhang T, et al. Low-intensity pulsed ultrasound promotes chondrogenesis of mesenchymal stem cells via regulation of autophagy. Stem Cell Res Ther 2019;10(1):41.

140. Liu DD, Ullah M, Concepcion W, et al. The role of ultrasound in enhancing mesenchymal stromal cell-based therapies. Stem Cells Transl Med 2020;9(8): 850–66.

141. Alvarez L. Extracorporeal shockwave therapy for musculoskeletal pathologies. Vet Clin North Am Small Anim Pract 2022;52(4):1033–42.

142. Becker W, Kowaleski MP, McCarthy RJ, et al. Extracorporeal shockwave therapy for shoulder lameness in dogs. J Am Anim Hosp Assoc 2015;51(1):15–9.

143. Gallagher A, Cross AR, Sepulveda G. The effect of shock wave therapy on patellar ligament desmitis after tibial plateau leveling osteotomy. Vet Surg 2012;41(4):482–5.

144. Leeman JJ, Shaw KK, Mison MB, et al. Extracorporeal shockwave therapy and therapeutic exercise for supraspinatus and biceps tendinopathies in 29 dogs. Vet Rec 2016;179(15):385.

145. Dahlberg J, Fitch G, Evans RB, et al. The evaluation of extracorporeal shockwave therapy in naturally occurring osteoarthritis of the stifle joint in dogs. Vet Comp Orthop Traumatol 2005;18(3):147–52.

146. Kersh KD, McClure SR, Van Sickle D, et al. The evaluation of extracorporeal shock wave therapy on collagenase induced superficial digital flexor tendonitis. Vet Comp Orthop Traumatol 2006;19(2):99–105.

147. Millis, DL, Drum, M, Whitlock D. Treatment of elbow arthritis with extracorporeal shock wave therapy. 2010 IAVRPT Symposium.

148. Kieves NR, MacKay CS, Adducci K, et al. High energy focused shock wave therapy accelerates bone healing. A blinded, prospective, randomized canine clinical trial. Vet Comp Orthop Traumatol 2015;28(6):425–32.

149. Seabaugh KA, Thoresen M, Giguère S. Extracorporeal shockwave therapy increases growth factor release from equine platelet-rich plasma In Vitro. Front Vet Sci 2017;4:205.

150. Facon-Poroszewska M, Kiełbowicz Z, Prządka P. Influence of radial pressure wave therapy (rpwt) on collagenase-induced Achilles tendinopathy treated with platelet rich plasma and autologous adipose derived stem cells. Pol J Vet Sci 2019;22(4):743–51.

151. Su W, Lin Y, Wang G, et al. Zhongguo Xiu Fu Chong Jian Wai Ke Za Zhi 2019; 33(12):1527–31.

152. Chang CY, Chen LC, Chou YC, et al. The effectiveness of platelet-rich plasma and radial extracorporeal shock wave compared with platelet-rich plasma in the treatment of moderate carpal tunnel syndrome. Pain Med 2020;21(8): 1668–75.

153. Zhang H, Li ZL, Yang F, et al. Radial shockwave treatment promotes human mesenchymal stem cell self-renewal and enhances cartilage healing. Stem Cell Res Ther 2018;9(1):54.

154. Zhang J, Kang N, Yu X, et al. Radial Extracorporeal Shock Wave Therapy Enhances the Proliferation and Differentiation of Neural Stem Cells by Notch, PI3K/AKT, and Wnt/β-catenin Signaling. Sci Rep 2017;7(1):15321.

155. Rinella L, Marano F, Paletto L, et al. Extracorporeal shock waves trigger tenogenic differentiation of human adipose-derived stem cells. Connect Tissue Res 2018;59(6):561–73.

156. Priglinger E, Schuh CMAP, Steffenhagen C, et al. Improvement of adipose tissue-derived cells by low-energy extracorporeal shock wave therapy. Cytotherapy 2017;19(9):1079–95.
157. Alshihri A, Niu W, Kämmerer PW, et al. The effects of shock wave stimulation of mesenchymal stem cells on proliferation, migration, and differentiation in an injectable gelatin matrix for osteogenic regeneration. J Tissue Eng Regen Med 2020;14(11):1630–40.
158. Hsu CC, Cheng JH, Wang CJ, et al. Shockwave therapy combined with autologous adipose-derived mesenchymal stem cells is better than with human umbilical cord wharton's jelly-derived mesenchymal stem cells on knee osteoarthritis. Int J Mol Sci 2020;21(4):1217.
159. Salcedo-Jiménez R, Koenig JB, Lee OJ, et al. Extracorporeal shock wave therapy enhances the *in vitro* metabolic activity and differentiation of equine umbilical cord blood mesenchymal stromal cells [published correction appears in front Vet Sci. 2022 Jan 28;9:840356]. Front Vet Sci 2020;7:554306.
160. Raabe O, Shell K, Goessl A, et al. Effect of extracorporeal shock wave on proliferation and differentiation of equine adipose tissue-derived mesenchymal stem cells in vitro. Am J Stem Cells 2013;2(1):62–73.
161. Weihs AM, Fuchs C, Teuschl AH, et al. Shock wave treatment enhances cell proliferation and improves wound healing by ATP release-coupled extracellular signal-regulated kinase (ERK) activation. J Biol Chem 2014;289(39):27090–104.
162. Schuh CM, Heher P, Weihs AM, et al. In vitro extracorporeal shock wave treatment enhances stemness and preserves multipotency of rat and human adipose-derived stem cells. Cytotherapy 2014;16(12):1666–78.
163. Suhr F, Delhasse Y, Bungartz G, et al. Cell biological effects of mechanical stimulations generated by focused extracorporeal shock wave applications on cultured human bone marrow stromal cells. Stem Cell Res 2013;11(2):951–64.
164. Cheng JH, Wang CJ, Chou WY, et al. Comparison efficacy of ESWT and Wharton's jelly mesenchymal stem cell in early osteoarthritis of rat knee. Am J Transl Res 2019;11(2):586–98.

Management of Injuries in Agility Dogs

Arielle Pechette Markley, DVM, cVMA, CVPP, CCRT, DAIPM*

KEYWORDS

- Sports medicine • Agility • Rehabilitation • Soft tissue injury • Biomechanics
- Lameness • Fitness

KEY POINTS

- Injuries are common in agility dogs, ranging from 32% to 42% based on five retrospective studies. The most common injuries in agility dogs are shoulder injuries (biceps tendinopathy, medial shoulder instability, and supraspinatus tendinopathy), iliopsoas strains, and back injuries.
- Risk factors for these injuries are complex and not well known. Border Collies seem to be at a higher risk of injury compared with other breeds. Increased body weight in relation to dog height has been correlated with increased risk for several injuries in agility dogs, including shoulder, digit, and stifle injuries.
- Treatment of injuries and rehabilitation planning relies on accurate diagnosis of the injury. Time to return to sport can be prolonged and prognosis to return to sport varies based on injury location and type.

INTRODUCTION

Canine agility is a physically demanding sport that requires the dog to navigate a complex predetermined course of obstacles within a certain timeframe and without incurring errors. The sport of canine agility has increased in popularity over the last decade, increasing from 870,603 entries in 2009 to 1,202,711 in 2019 for American Kennel Club hosted agility trials alone.[1] As the popularity of the sport has increased, so has the competitiveness, speed, and difficulty of course design. As the sport of agility has grown, so has the field of sports medicine and rehabilitation. Agility handlers are a very dedicated client population and are quick to seek veterinary and complementary care for their canine athletes, both for preventative purposes and when injuries are sustained. It is important that the veterinary practitioner understand the physical demands of the sport of agility and the common injury patterns seen in agility dogs to best diagnose and treat injuries in this population. Unfortunately, there is a lack of prospective

Department of Clinical Sciences, Sports Medicine and Rehabilitation, The Ohio State University College of Veterinary Medicine, 601 Vernon L Tharp Street, Columbus, Ohio 43210, USA
* Corresponding author.
E-mail address: Markley.125@osu.edu

Vet Clin Small Anim 53 (2023) 829–844
https://doi.org/10.1016/j.cvsm.2023.02.012   **vetsmall.theclinics.com**
0195-5616/23/© 2023 Elsevier Inc. All rights reserved.

research on agility injuries, risk factors for injury, and rehabilitation therapy for the canine athlete. Therefore, much of our knowledge and current recommendations are based on retrospective studies and data extrapolated from human and equine medicine.

INCIDENCE OF INJURIES IN AGILITY DOGS

Over the past decade, there has been an increase in awareness of agility injuries and interest in profiling common injuries and determining potential risk factors for injury. There have been multiple retrospective surveys performed in the past two decades that provide insight into common agility injuries and risk factors.[2–8] The most significant limitation of all the current data on agility injuries is the fact that the information was gathered via owner-reported, retrospective survey methods. There are currently no published prospective studies on agility dog injuries. Each of the surveys used different populations, outcome assessments, and survey design, thereby providing varying snapshots into agility dog health and injuries (**Table 1**).

Surveys report an injury rate in agility dogs ranging from 32% to 42%. However, owing to the limitations of survey design, it is unknown how many of these injuries are a direct result of participation in agility. Not only are injuries common but also multiple injuries seem to be frequent. The recent 2019 survey by Pechette Markley and colleagues reported that 49% of injured dogs had more than one injury that kept them out of agility for over a week.[5] This is in contrast to the 2009 survey by Cullen and colleagues where only 27.6% of dogs had more than one injury.[3]

Unfortunately, it is impossible to determine whether the incidence of injuries in agility dogs has truly increased over the past decade or whether other factors, such as the

Table 1
Surveys of injury rates for dogs engaged in the sport of agility[2,3,5–7]

Author, Year	Data Collection Method/Sample	Outcome Measures	Injury Rate (n Injured/n Dogs)
Levy,[2] 2009	Mail and online survey distributed via Clean Run in 2005–2006; United States only	Injury during competition or practice in the 2 y	33% (529/1627)
Cullen,[3] 2013	Online survey distributed in 2009; 84% North American	Any agility training- or competition-related injury	32% (1209/3801)
Evanow,[6] 2021	In person survey at Midwest/Northeast U.S. agility trials in 2015 (dog competing at trial)	Ever injured while participating in or training for agility	28% (142/500)
Pechette Markley,[5] 2021	Online survey distributed via social media in 2019; 71% North American; (dog alive and competed in past 3 y)	Any injury keeping dog out of agility practice or competition for over a week	42% (1958/4701)
Inkila,[7] 2022a	Online survey through Finnish Agility Association; Survey completed in 2020 (dog had to have competed in 2018 or 2019 and trained for agility in 2019)	Any previous agility-related injury; Agility-related injury in 2019	32% (278/864) any prior 14% (119/864) in 2019

growth of the specialty of sports medicine and rehabilitation and sports medicine education for veterinarians and handlers, have increased the awareness and diagnosis of injuries that were previously undiagnosed. Regardless, this population of athletes seems to have a high rate of injuries, so a thorough knowledge of common injuries is needed for the veterinary practitioner seeing agility dogs in their practice.

TYPES OF INJURIES IN AGILITY DOGS

The key to successful treatment and rehabilitation of injuries in agility dogs, particularly soft tissue injuries, is the accurate identification of affected structure(s) as well as the full assessment of the patient to identify secondary and compensatory changes. It is, therefore, helpful to know what injuries are commonly diagnosed in this patient population. Although there is variation between the survey methods in the current agility literature, there is a lot of overlap with regard to types of injuries commonly seen in agility dogs. All surveys have reported that shoulder and back injuries are the most commonly sustained, with iliopsoas muscle and digits also regularly reported (**Table 2**).[2,3,5–7] Of the known shoulder pathologies, biceps tendinopathy, medial shoulder instability (MSI), and supraspinatus tendinopathy are the most frequently reported.[5] Of iliopsoas muscle injuries, strains are most common.[5]

There are reported differences in injury rate and type of injury by both breed and geographic region.[5] Border Collies have been consistently reported to have the highest rate of injury across all surveys, even when breed is adjusted for in statistical models. Injury rate and type may vary by breed due to structural differences, genetic factors relating to injury predisposition, temperament differences, speed, and handler factors. Geographic differences in injury rate and type may be associated with differences in agility cultures (types of courses, surface, practice habits, and so forth), differences in dogs doing agility by country, different access to specialists/diagnostics, or differences in handlers who filled out the survey by country.

RISK FACTORS FOR INJURY

Identification of risk factors for injury is important for both prevention of injury and for adjusting training and competition strategies post-injury. However, risk factor analysis is complex. Using retrospective survey data further complicates data evaluation. To date, retrospective survey data is all that has been used in published risk factor studies. Many of the retrospective surveys have evaluated various risk factors including demographic risk factors and training and competition risk factors.[4,6–9]

Border Collies have been shown to have a higher risk of injury in adjusted models across multiple samples and surveys.[4–8] It is unknown why Border Collies have an increased risk of injury compared with other breeds but proposed causes include genetics, conformation, speed of runs performed, and high-drive temperament. Speed has been postulated to be a risk factor for increased injury in racing greyhounds.[10] In human athletes, there is an increased risk of muscle injury with both high speed and the behavioral tendency to override pain and keep performing.[11] It is possible that the combination of high speed of the Border Collie breed and the high drive for work both increase the risk of injury and also delay identification of injury until that injury is more severe.

Other risk factor correlations are less clear and not as consistent across studies. Handler experience seems to play a role in injury risk, with dogs of more experienced handlers having a decreased risk of injury and dogs of less experienced handlers having an increased risk of injury.[4,8,9] Competition at high level seems to be associated with increased injury risk.[6,8] Another factor which has been associated with increased injury in multiple studies is increased weight as compared with height.[4,9,12,13] There

Table 2
Reported percentage of injured dogs with injury to common anatomic locations by survey[2,3,5–7]

Author, Year	Overall Rate	Shoulder	Back	Percentage of Injured Dogs Reporting Injury to the Region Iliopsoas muscle	Stifle	Digits
Levy,[2] 2009	33%	20%	18%	Not directly reported: 6% thigh; 6% hip	12%	6%
Cullen,[3] 2013	32%	23%	19%	Not directly reported; 12% upper thigh	11%	13%
Evanow,[6] 2021	28%	17%	18%	13%	8%	12%
Pechette Markley,[5] 2021	42%	30%	17% lumbosacral; 13% thoracic	19%	13%	18%
Inkila,[7,71] 2022a,b, 2019 injuries	14%	13% shoulder; 13% scapular region	19%	Not directly reported; 11% thigh; 4% groin	3%	10% (front limb), 5% (hind limb)

are many other variables that have been proposed as risk factors for injury such as jump height, contact obstacle behaviors (stopped vs running contacts), weave training, surface, frequency of training and competition, but correlations are not well known based on the currently available retrospective data.[8,14]

Risk factors for more specific injuries and anatomic locations have been evaluated both in general surveys and in targeted injury surveys. These evaluations have the same limitations of being retrospective in nature, but typically have the additional limitation of smaller sample size. Injury-specific surveys have investigated risk factors for digit injury and cranial cruciate ligament rupture.[12,13] The broader injury surveys have also analyzed data to examine risk factors associated with shoulder, stifle, lumbosacral, and iliopsoas injury.[15–19] The most consistent finding was that heavier dogs, in relation to height, had an increased risk of digit injury, general stifle injury, cranial cruciate ligament rupture, and shoulder injury. Other risk factors were observed but varied by injury type and anatomic location.

Although understanding the risk factors for injury is critical for determining injury prevention and treatment strategies, many of the variables for injury risk remain unclear and will require long-term prospective longitudinal studies to elucidate factors of clinical relevance. Based on the currently available data, it seems that Border Collies have a consistently higher risk of injury, which increases the index of suspicion for injury in this population when performance changes are noted. Also of clinical relevance, it seems that increased weight in relation to height increases risk of multiple types of injury, including digit, shoulder, and stifle injury. As this is a modifiable possible risk factor, unlike many of the other agility-related variables, educating agility clients regarding the importance of weight management should be a top priority in the discussion of injury prevention.

CLINICS CARE POINTS

- Maintaining an ideal body condition seems to reduce the risk of multiple agility-related injuries. Therefore, it is imperative that the practitioner discuss weight management with all agility dog owners.

BIOMECHANICS OF AGILITY

Understanding the movement patterns and forces placed on a dog's body during agility is critical to understanding injury patterns, potential injury prevention strategies, and tailoring rehabilitation and return to sport plans to the demands of agility. A number of studies have been performed to evaluate biomechanics in agility dogs. Current studies have evaluated both kinematics (movement) and kinetics (forces) for some jumping-specific tasks and A-frame performance. No studies have evaluated the dog walk, teeter, tunnel, varying jump approaches/exits, course design, surface, or effect of handling on biomechanics. A full review of agility biomechanics is beyond the scope of this article; however, key points as related to possible injury are discussed below.

Jumping biomechanics are different between advanced and beginner dogs. Beginner dogs have lower forelimb stiffness and increased compression when landing, which may increase the risk of soft tissue injuries, particularly of the shoulder.[20,21] Therefore, clinically, this may provide an avenue for injury prevention through jump-specific training and conditioning as well as monitoring training progress. Higher jump heights have been shown to increase peak vertical force and landing angles, with forces in the forelimbs incurring up to 4.5 times the bodyweight.[22] Both jump height and distance between jumps have been shown to affect joint angulation, speed, and jump trajectory.[23–27] The correlation between these biomechanical alterations and injury remains unknown.

A study by Cullen and colleagues used electromyography to evaluate the muscular activation in the biceps brachii, supraspinatus, infraspinatus, and triceps brachii muscles during jumping and A-frame agility tasks. [28] This study found that, between the two agility tasks, triceps and biceps activation were significantly higher when jumping, and supraspinatus activation was highest when leaving the A-frame. Overall, the jump task was consistently the most demanding across all four forelimb muscles. This high degree of muscle activation required for jumping combined with the frequency of jumps on each agility course could contribute to injuries in this population of athletes.

Several studies have evaluated kinetics and kinematics of A-frame performance.[29–33] These studies found that decreasing the A-frame angle of incline did not significantly decrease carpal extension angle but decreased propulsive force and time in propulsion, that carpal braces did not significantly reduce carpal extension during A-frame, or jump, and performance, and that joint range of motion varies based on the different phases of A-frame performance.[29–31,33] Currently, no published studies describe the biomechanics of weave performance, though one recent study defined and evaluated paw placement patterns in dogs completing the weave obstacle.[34] Again, the correlation between these findings and injury risk and prevention is unknown, and further studies are needed to make clinical recommendations regarding training and performance of these obstacles.

COMMON PERFORMANCE PROBLEMS

Although many of the soft tissue injuries diagnosed in agility dogs present with lameness, the lameness may be only very mild or intermittent. In the cases of less severe injury or in dogs with high drive, lameness may not be appreciable. In these patients, injury may only be indicated by performance-related changes noted by handlers. Some of the commonly reported performance issues include decreased speed on course, popping out of weave poles, missed weave pole entries, refusing contact obstacles or change of performance on the contact obstacle, refusing certain lines or direction of turns, and not changing lead legs as appropriate. Problems with jumping are also often reported. Jumping issues can include refusing jumps, knocking bars, stutter stepping before takeoff, and change in jump style or trajectory. One of the most reported changes in jump style that is often associated with injury is a change from jumping with the pelvic limbs extended to jumping with the hips flexed and pelvic limbs tucked under the body during the jump. Reviewing agility training and competition videos in slow motion can aid in identifying subtle performance changes. Although some of these changes may lead to suspicion of certain injuries, many are nonspecific. All performance problems should indicate a need for a thorough physical evaluation of the patient by an experienced veterinarian.

CLINICS CARE POINTS

- Agility dogs presenting with an injury may not have an appreciable lameness or history of lameness. It is critical for the practitioner to consider the handler's perception of the performance problem even if it seems minor.

COMMON AGILITY INJURIES
Shoulder Region

Shoulder injuries are the most commonly reported injury in agility dogs. Based on a recent survey, shoulder injuries represent about 30% of the injuries in agility dogs.[5]

Of the known specific shoulder injuries, biceps tendinopathy, MSI, and supraspinatus tendinopathy are most frequently described.[5]

Biceps brachii tendinopathy

Biceps tendinopathy is most often seen in large-breed, active dogs, but can be seen in agility dogs of any age or breed. Biceps tendinopathy represents about 19% of known reported shoulder injuries in agility dogs.[5] The lameness may be acute, chronic, or intermittent. Pain may be noted on direct palpation of the biceps tendon or muscle and is more often noted on "biceps stretch test." The biceps stretch test is defined as full flexion of the shoulder with concurrent extension of the elbow. If complete rupture of the biceps is present, then there is an increased range of motion on elbow extension relative to the extension present in a dog with without rupture during biceps test with a significant change in end feel to an absence of muscle resistance. Radiographs should be performed to rule out other pathology and may show degenerative changes in the bicipital groove and mineralization of the tendon within the bicipital groove (though mineralization may not be clinically significant and is not a good indicator of active biceps pathology).[35] Although MRI has been shown to be sensitive for identifying biceps pathology, musculoskeletal ultrasound seems to have more clinical usefulness in both initial diagnosis and in monitoring progression of disease and/or response to treatment.[36–40] Retrospective studies have reported improvement in biceps tendinopathy with shockwave therapy and rehabilitation exercise therapy.[41] Orthobiologic therapy is often used in the treatment of biceps tendinopathy, but there are no studies evaluating this use in canine patients. However, orthobiologics have shown positive results in human patients with biceps tendonitis and rotator cuff injuries.[42,43] Surgical management, such as biceps tenotomy or tenodesis, are also proposed options for cases with severe pathology or those that fail conservative management. [44–46]

Supraspinatus tendinopathy

Supraspinatus tendinopathy most often occurs in medium to large-breed active dogs and presents as a chronic, intermittent thoracic limb lameness that is unresponsive to rest and nonsteroidal anti-inflammatory drugs.[47] Full shoulder flexion is often painful, as it stretches the supraspinatus. Some dogs show a pain response to direct palpation of the supraspinatus. Isolated supraspinatus tendinopathy rarely occurs and is more often seen concurrently with other pathologies such as biceps tendinopathy and MSI or concurrently with elbow osteoarthritis.[47] Ultrasound is the most cost-effective imaging modality and can differentiate between supraspinatus tendinopathy and biceps tendinopathy.[38,40] Retrospective studies have reported improvement in supraspinatus tendinopathy with orthobiologic therapy, shockwave therapy, and rehabilitation exercise therapy.[41,48,49]

Medial shoulder instability/syndrome

MSI is caused by pathology of the medial structures of the shoulder joint. The disruption of the medial glenohumeral ligament, subscapularis tendon, or both may be involved. MSI is often seen in middle-aged working and sporting dogs. Presentation may be as mild as decreased sport performance or as severe as non-weight-bearing lameness if there is significant disruption with subluxation. Examination findings can be nonspecific with shoulder pain on range of motion, decreased shoulder extension, and muscle atrophy. Pain on abduction and increased abduction angles can be present but are not necessarily definitive for the diagnosis of shoulder instability. Studies evaluating abduction angles as a diagnostic tool for MSI have had conflicting results, and it is not recommended to use this test as a definitive diagnosis for

MSI, but it can be useful when coupled with other diagnostics.[50–52] Abduction angle, therefore, may provide an index for suspicion but should not be used for definitive diagnosis. Arthroscopy is the gold standard diagnostic for MSI.[53] Treatment for MSI depends on the degree of injury and which structures are damaged. Nonsurgical treatment usually involves the use of a shoulder stabilization system (hobbles) and rehabilitation therapy. More severe instability typically requires surgical reconstruction of ligaments with no specific procedure having been shown to be superior.[54]

Iliopsoas tendinopathy

The iliopsoas muscle is formed by the psoas major and iliacus muscles. The main functions of the iliopsoas are flexion of the hip, adduction, and external rotation of the femur, as well as core stabilization and flexion of the lumbar spine. In a study by Nielsen and Pluhar, the iliopsoas muscle was reported to be the most common muscle strained in the pelvic limb.[55] In a recent study by Pechette Markley and colleagues of 4701 dogs competing in agility competitions, iliopsoas injuries were the second most commonly reported injury with 380 total dogs reporting this injury (19.4% of all injured dogs).[5,15] It is thought that iliopsoas injuries can occur as a primary injury either as a result of acute stretch-induced injury or repetitive microtrauma, or as a secondary injury due underlying orthopedic or neurologic pathology. Thorough examination is essential to ensure that any underlying pathology is identified. Traumatic incidents that result in active eccentric muscle contraction, such as slipping into a splay-legged position, jumping out of a vehicle, agility training, or rough-housing with other dogs, are often suspected in precipitating acute lameness.

Dogs with iliopsoas strains commonly present with a history ranging from a subtle intermittent offloading of the hindlimb to significant unilateral hindlimb lameness that is exacerbated with activity. These dogs commonly have reluctance to jump, and agility dogs often demonstrate performance issues, such as knocking bars and slowing in the weave poles.

On gait evaluation, dogs will often have a shortened stride with reluctance to fully extend the hip. On physical examination, these patients may have pain with hip extension that is similar to patients with hip dysplasia. It is important to attempt to separate this discomfort from joint discomfort, or lumbosacral pain as the lumbosacral region can easily undergo motion when extending the hip joint. Discomfort and spasm may be noted on the direct palpation of the iliopsoas at its insertion on the lesser trochanter. Pain and spasm may also be noted when stretching the myotendinous unit by either placing the hip in extension with abduction or by simultaneous extension of the hip with internal rotation. Pain can also be elicited with digital pressure over the muscle body cranioventral to the wing of the ilium and at its insertion on the lesser trochanter.

Commonly no radiographic changes are seen with iliopsoas injuries; however, occasional enthesophytes are noted at the lesser trochanter. Despite this, radiographs should be made as they can be useful to rule out concurrent hip, lumbosacral, and stifle pathology. Ultrasonography is usually the diagnostic of choice, and the grading scales based on ultrasonographic appearance have been described in the literature.[56] MRI has been reported to be sensitive in detecting iliopsoas pathology, but due to cost and requirement for general anesthesia, MRI may not be as practical, except in cases where evaluating for lumbosacral disease is a priority.[57,58] The ability of ultrasound to grade the strain may also be useful for determining treatment, though no prospective studies evaluating treatment protocols have been published.

Treatment involves addressing any concurrent or underlying conditions as well as treating the iliopsoas injury itself. In general, medical management for iliopsoas tendinopathy involves exercise restriction, pharmaceuticals as indicated (Non-steroidal anti-inflammatories, methocarbamol, gabapentin), rehabilitation therapy once to twice a week, and a home exercise program. For milder cases, rehabilitation therapy generally includes photobiomodulation therapy, manual/massage therapy, pulsed electromagnetic field therapy (PEMF), transcutaneous electrical nerve stimulation, and home exercise plans. In more severe cases, orthobiologics and extracorporeal shockwave therapy are used, in addition to the other listed modalities. Exercise plans focus on core strength and isometric muscle engagement, progressing to concentric and eccentric muscle engagement. Underwater treadmill is not recommended in the initial healing phase and is usually introduced at about 8 weeks. Timeline for recovery heavily depends on the grade of injury and concurrent musculoskeletal injuries or conditions, but 2 to 4 months of rehabilitation therapy, followed by 2 to 3 months of conditioning/sport-retraining is not uncommon. In rare cases, surgical release has been reported and should be reserved for refractory cases.[58]

LESS COMMON AGILITY INJURIES
Carpus

Abductor pollicus longus
The abductor pollicus longus originates from the lateral surface of the radius and ulna, as well as the interosseous membrane, and tracts medially to insert on the proximal aspect of the first metacarpal bone. The muscle is an abductor of the first digit, an adductor of the carpus, and is a medial stabilizer of the carpus. Dogs frequently present with a chronic, mild forelimb lameness and have visible and palpable firm swelling medial to the distal radius. Radiographs often show enthesopathy and bony proliferation along the radial sulcus. Musculoskeletal ultrasound may be useful in evaluating for fluid accumulation, thickening of the abductor pollicis longus tendon, and thickening of the abductor pollicis longus synovial sheath.[59,60] Medical and surgical treatment options have been described in the literature. Medical treatment usually includes injection with a corticosteroid or an orthobiologic, photobiomodulation therapy, and extracorporeal shockwave therapy. Surgical treatment to release is rarely needed.

Flexor carpi ulnaris tendinopathy
The flexor carpi ulnaris (FCU) is made up of two bellies (the ulnar head and the humeral head), which converge into one tendon that inserts on the accessory carpal bone. On examination, a firm swelling/thickening can be palpated at the insertion point on the accessory carpal bone and pain may be elicited on hyperextension of the carpus. Although radiographs may show soft tissue swelling or calcification, musculoskeletal ultrasound is the diagnostic modality of choice.[60] No studies are available regarding best treatment protocols, but photobiomodulation therapy, intratendinous injections of an orthobiologic, and extracorporeal shockwave therapy can be used. There are reports of FCU injury causing hyperextension of the carpus. These cases may require surgical intervention.[61]

Accessoriometacarpal ligament desmitis
The accessoriometacarpal ligament originates on the lateral aspect of the accessory carpal bone and inserts on the base of the fifth metacarpal bone. Avulsion of this ligament is reported in racing Greyhounds, though cases of sprains and desmitis are seen in active sporting dogs such as hunting dogs and agility dogs. Mild, sometimes intermittent, lameness is noted and is often worse after activity. On examination, firm swelling can be palpated along the lateral aspect of the carpus, between the accessory carpal bone and fifth metacarpal bone. Pain is usually present

on flexion of the carpus, and the range of motion on flexion is often reduced. Musculoskeletal ultrasound is the best imaging modality, though radiographs can show enthesopathy and soft tissue swelling in the region. No studies are available regarding best treatment protocols, but photobiomodulation therapy, intraligamentous injections (orthobiologic or corticosteroid), and shockwave therapy can be used.

PELVIC LIMB
Gastrocnemius Musculotendinopathy

The gastrocnemius muscle consists of lateral and medial heads, which arise from the lateral and medial supracondylar tuberosity of the femur. Both heads contain a sesamoid bone named fabella. The muscle bellies combine distally to create the gastrocnemius tendon, which inserts on the calcaneus. Musculotendinopathy of the lateral head of the gastrocnemius muscle is a rare condition that is most commonly reported in herding and sporting dogs. Lameness can be mild and intermittent to severe. Dogs may have a shortened stride with a skip in their gait, as they often resist extension of the stifle and flexion of the tarsus, actions that stretch the gastrocnemius muscle. Dogs may be painful on stifle palpation, and care should be made to differentiate the pain from that of stifle pathology such as cranial cruciate ligament rupture. Dogs are often painful specifically on palpation of the lateral fabella and may be painful on stifle extension with concurrent tarsal flexion. Radiographs are often abnormal, and findings can include significant osteophyte formation and dystrophic mineralization around the lateral fabella that can give the appearance of a fragmented fabella, and periosteal reaction on the caudal aspect of the femur. MRI and musculoskeletal ultrasound can also be used to identify the degree of pathology.[62,63] Medical management includes exercise restriction, photobiomodulation therapy, orthobiologics, extracorporeal shockwave, and PEMF, though no studies have prospectively evaluated treatment protocols.

Rehabilitation, Conditioning/Reconditioning

The standard rehabilitation principles apply to all soft tissue injuries in agility dogs. Rehabilitation of shoulder injuries and other soft tissue injuries have been previously described; however, prospective studies in dogs are lacking.[64–67] There are no studies specifically evaluating rehabilitation protocols for treatment of injury in agility dogs. Once healing is complete; however, the rehabilitation goals must be adjusted to address reconditioning and sport-specific training. Strength exercises must be targeted and focus on the movements needed for agility performance. No studies have been performed to evaluate sport-specific training or conditioning programs in agility dogs, and much research is needed to determine the best protocols for treatment and prevention of injury in these athletes.

Prognosis and Return to Sport

Prognosis for return to sport is often a primary concern of agility handlers as their dogs recover from injuries. Unfortunately, there are limited studies evaluating return to agility after injury. In a survey by Tomlinson and colleagues, 67% of dogs returned to competing in agility, 11% returned to training but not competition, and 22% did not return to sport. Of the dogs that returned to competition, 47% of them jumped a lower competition jump height after returning. There was a higher rate of return to competition in dogs that underwent conservative management for their injury compared with surgical management (70% vs 61%).[68]

Owing to the small sample sizes for most of the individual injuries, conclusions could not be made regarding prognosis for return sport in the majority of cases. However, dogs that underwent stifle surgery were less likely to return to competition (52%) and were more likely to decrease jump height class if they returned to competing. A separate retrospective study looked specifically at dogs returning to agility after tibial plateau leveling osteotomy and found that 65% of the 31 dogs returned to competition.[69] Although these data provide insight into return to agility after stifle injury and surgery, overall little is known about return to agility with the more common agility injuries.

A recent study by Entani and colleagues evaluated the use of serial ultrasonography in the assessment of soft-tissue shoulder injury recovery with rehabilitation therapy and determination of time to return to sport.[39] The most affected structures included biceps brachii, supraspinatus, and infraspinatus muscles and tendons. Rehabilitation therapy in these patients included photobiomodulation therapy, therapeutic ultrasound, range of motion exercises, and underwater treadmill therapy. At 2 months, 78% of patients had no apparent lameness on subjective evaluation, but none had ultrasonographic evidence of healing. At 4 months, 44% of dogs still had lesions present on ultrasound, so return to sport was delayed an additional 6 weeks. At 6 months, 70% of dogs had minimal ultrasound changes that persisted but all were back doing agility training, so the changes were proposed to be clinically insignificant.[39] The slow resolution of ultrasound changes in this study is in contrast to the studies on orthobiologic therapies. One study reported significant improvement in supraspinatus tendon size, fiber pattern, and echogenicity at 90 days after bone marrow aspirate concentrate - platelet rich plasma (BMAC-PRP) treatment[48] and another that indicated that 96% of dogs returned to sport 4 months after adipose-derived progenitor cells - platelet rich plasma (ADPC-PRP) treatment.[49] Given the variability in ultrasound improvement and return to sport seen, prospective studies on treatment protocols for shoulder injuries in agility dogs are needed before definitive recommendations can be made.

In a recent conference abstract, based on the data from a retrospective survey, agility handlers reported a return to competition and training within a month most frequently for metacarpus, carpus, and antebrachium injuries and least frequently for stifle, tarsus, iliopsoas, and tibia injuries. The longest return to competition and training was reported for stifle injuries, with 25% of dogs taking greater than 6 months to return and another 21% reporting that the dog was officially retired from agility. The rate of retirement was generally low for most locations being less than 10% for all categories, except the hip (10%), stifle (21%), and tarsus (18%). Only 34 dogs had a tarsus injury reported, but a long return to competition time was observed for these dogs as well (21% > 6 months; 18% officially retired).[70]

CONCLUSION: REHABILITATION CONSIDERATIONS FOR AGILITY DOGS

Agility is a physically demanding sport and injuries are common. An understanding of the common clinical presentations, most frequent injuries, risk factors for injury, and the demands of the sport is critical when seeing this population of patients in practice. Shoulder injuries along with other soft tissue injuries including iliopsoas strains are commonly seen. The Border Collie seems to be at higher risk of developing agility-related injuries. Discussion regarding their risk of injury should proactively take place with owners. The key to rehabilitation of the agility dog is accurate and expedient diagnosis of the injury, which often involves advanced diagnostics such as musculoskeletal ultrasound, arthroscopy, and/or MRI. Identification of the specific injury allows for prompt, targeted treatment, and serial monitoring of treatment success. The goal for these patients is to return them safely to sport and minimize the risk of reinjury. Time to return to sport can be prolonged and varies based on injury location and type. No prospective studies are currently available evaluating agility dog injuries, risk factors, or best treatment and rehabilitation protocols. Future prospective studies will be beneficial for providing better injury prevention and treatment for canine agility athletes.

DISCLOSURE

The author has no conflicts of interest to disclose.

REFERENCES

1. Carrie DeYoung, Director of Agility, American Kennel Club. Personal Commun 2020.
2. Levy M, Hall C, Trentacosta N, et al. A preliminary retrospective survey of injuries occurring in dogs participating in canine agility. Vet Comp Orthop Traumatol 2009;22(4):321–4.
3. Cullen KL, Dickey JP, Bent LR, et al. Internet-based survey of the nature and perceived causes of injury to dogs participating in agility training and competition events. J Am Vet Med Assoc 2013;243(7):1010–8.
4. Cullen KL, Dickey JP, Bent LR, et al. Survey-based analysis of risk factors for injury among dogs participating in agility training and competition events. J Am Vet Med Assoc 2013;243(7):1019–24.
5. Pechette Markley A, Shoben AB, Kieves NR. Internet-based survey of the frequency and types of orthopedic conditions and injuries experienced by dogs competing in agility. J Am Vet Med Assoc 2021;259(9):1001–8.
6. Evanow JA, VanDeventer G, Dinallo G, et al. Internet survey of participant demographics and risk factors for injury in competitive agility dogs. VCOT Open 2021; 4(2):e92–8.
7. Inkilä L, Hyytiäinen HK, Hielm-Björkman A, et al. Part II of Finnish Agility Dog Survey: Agility-Related Injuries and Risk Factors for Injury in Competition-Level Agility Dogs. Animals (Basel) 2022;12(3). https://doi.org/10.3390/ani12030227.
8. Pechette Markley A, Shoben AB, Kieves NR. Internet survey of risk factors associated with training and competition in dogs competing in agility competitions. Front Vet Sci 2021;8:791617.
9. Sundby AE, Pechette Markley A, Shoben AB, et al. Internet survey evaluation of demographic risk factors for injury in canine agility athletes. Front Vet Sci 2022;9: 869702.
10. Sicard GK, Short K, Manley PA. A survey of injuries at five greyhound racing tracks. J Small Anim Pract 1999;40(9):428–32.
11. Hoskins W, Pollard H. The management of hamstring injury–Part 1: Issues in diagnosis. Man Ther 2005;10(2):96–107.
12. Sellon DC, Martucci K, Wenz JR, et al. A survey of risk factors for digit injuries among dogs training and competing in agility events. J Am Vet Med Assoc 2018;252(1):75–83.
13. Sellon DC, Marcellin-Little DJ. Risk factors for cranial cruciate ligament rupture in dogs participating in canine agility. BMC Vet Res 2022;18(1):39.
14. Jimenez IA, Canapp SO, Percival ML. Internet-based survey evaluating the impact of ground substrate on injury and performance in canine agility athletes. Front Vet Sci 2022;9. https://doi.org/10.3389/fvets.2022.1025331.

15. Fry LM, Kieves NR, Shoben AB, et al. Internet survey evaluation of iliopsoas injury in dogs participating in agility competitions. Front Vet Sci 2022;9:930450.

16. Pechette Markley A, Shoben AB, Kieves NR. Risk Factors Associated with Lumbosacral Injury in Dogs Competing in Agility Competitions. Scientific Presentation Abstracts. 2021 ACVS Surgery Summit October 7-9, Chicago, Illinois. Vet Surg 2021. https://doi.org/10.1111/vsu.13706.

17. Pechette Markley A, Shoben AB, Kieves NR. Risk Factors Associated with Iliopsoas Injury in Dogs Competing in Agility Competitions. Scientific Presentation Abstracts. 2021 ACVS Surgery Summit October 7-9, Chicago, Illinois. Vet Surg 2021. https://doi.org/10.1111/vsu.13706.

18. Kieves NR, Shoben AB, Pechette Markley A. Risk Factors for the Development of Stifle Injuries in Canine Agility Athletes. Scientific Presentation Abstracts. 2021 ACVS Surgery Summit October 7-9, Chicago, Illinois. Vet Surg 2021. https://doi.org/10.1111/vsu.13706.

19. Kieves N.R., Shoben A.B., Pechette Markley A., Risk Factors for the Development of Shoulder Injuries in Dogs Competing in Agility. Scientific Presentation Abstracts. 2021 ACVS Surgery Summit October 7-9, Chicago, IL, Vet Surg, 2021, https://doi.org/10.1111/vsu.13706.

20. Söhnel K, Rode C, de Lussanet MHE, et al. Limb dynamics in agility jumps of beginner and advanced dogs. J Exp Biol 2020;223(Pt 7). https://doi.org/10.1242/jeb.202119.

21. Söhnel K, Andrada E, de Lussanet MHE, et al. Single limb dynamics of jumping turns in dogs. Res Vet Sci 2021;140:69–78.

22. Pfau T, Garland de Rivaz A, Brighton S, et al. Kinetics of jump landing in agility dogs. Vet J 2011;190(2):278–83.

23. Alcock J, Birch E, Boyd J. Effect of jumping style on the performance of large and medium elite agility dogs. Comp Exerc Physiol 2015;11(3):145–50.

24. Birch E, Carter A, Boyd J. An examination of jump kinematics in dogs over increasing hurdle heights. Comp Exerc Physiol 2016;12(2):91–8.

25. Birch E, Boyd J, Doyle G, et al. Small and medium agility dogs alter their kinematics when the distance between hurdles differs. Comp Exerc Physiol 2015;11(2):75–8.

26. Birch E, Leśniak K. Effect of fence height on joint angles of agility dogs. Vet J 2013;198(Suppl 1):e99–102.

27. Birch E, Boyd J, Doyle G, et al. The effects of altered distances between obstacles on the jump kinematics and apparent joint angulations of large agility dogs. Vet J 2015;204(2):174–8.

28. Cullen KL, Dickey JP, Brown SHM, et al. The magnitude of muscular activation of four canine forelimb muscles in dogs performing two agility-specific tasks. BMC Vet Res 2017;13(1):68.

29. Appelgrein C, Glyde MR, Hosgood G, et al. Reduction of the A-Frame Angle of Incline does not Change the Maximum Carpal Joint Extension Angle in Agility Dogs Entering the A-Frame. Vet Comp Orthop Traumatol 2018;31(2):77–82.

30. Blake S, de Godoy RF. Kinematics and kinetics of dogs completing jump and A-frame exercises. Comp Exerc Physiol 2021;17(4):351–66.

31. Appelgrein C, Glyde MR, Hosgood G, et al. Kinetic Gait Analysis of Agility Dogs Entering the A-Frame. Vet Comp Orthop Traumatol 2019;32(2):97–103.

32. Williams JM, Jackson R, Phillips C, et al. The effect of the A-frame on forelimb kinematics in experienced and inexperienced agility dogs. Comp Exerc Physiol 2017;13(4):243–9.

33. Castilla A, Knotek B, Vitt M, et al. Carpal Extension Angles in Agility Dogs Exiting the A-Frame and Hurdle Jumps. Vet Comp Orthop Traumatol 2020;33(2):142–6.

34. Eicher LD, Markley AP, Shoben A, et al. Evaluation of variability in gait styles used by dogs completing weave poles in agility competition and its effect on completion of the obstacle. Front Vet Sci 2021;8:761493.

35. Muir P, Johnson KA. Supraspinatus and biceps brachii tendinopathy in dogs. J Small Anim Pract 1994;35(5):239–43.

36. Kramer M, Gerwing M, Sheppard C, et al. Ultrasonography for the diagnosis of diseases of the tendon and tendon sheath of the biceps brachii muscle. Vet Surg 2001;30(1):64–71.

37. Murphy SE, Ballegeer EA, Forrest LJ, et al. Magnetic resonance imaging findings in dogs with confirmed shoulder pathology. Vet Surg 2008;37(7):631–8.

38. Lassaigne CC, Boyer C, Sautier L, et al. Ultrasound of the normal canine supraspinatus tendon: comparison with gross anatomy and histology. Vet Rec 2020; 186(17):e14.

39. Entani MG, Franini A, Dragone L, et al. Efficacy of Serial Ultrasonographic Examinations in Predicting Return to Play in Agility Dogs with Shoulder Lameness. Animals (Basel) 2021;12(1). https://doi.org/10.3390/ani12010078.

40. Barella G, Lodi M, Faverzani S. Ultrasonographic findings of shoulder tenomuscular structures in symptomatic and asymptomatic dogs. J Ultrasound 2018;21(2):145–52.

41. Leeman JJ, Shaw KK, Mison MB, et al. Extracorporeal shockwave therapy and therapeutic exercise for supraspinatus and biceps tendinopathies in 29 dogs. Vet Rec 2016;179(15):385.

42. Sanli I, Morgan B, van Tilborg F, et al. Single injection of platelet-rich plasma (PRP) for the treatment of refractory distal biceps tendonitis: long-term results of a prospective multicenter cohort study. Knee Surg Sports Traumatol Arthrosc 2016;24(7):2308–12.

43. Xu W, Xue Q. Application of Platelet-Rich Plasma in Arthroscopic Rotator Cuff Repair: A Systematic Review and Meta-analysis. Orthop J Sports Med 2021; 9(7). https://doi.org/10.1177/23259671211016847. 23259671211016850.

44. Bergenhuyzen ALR, Vermote KAG, van Bree H, et al. Long-term follow-up after arthroscopic tenotomy for partial rupture of the biceps brachii tendon. Vet Comp Orthop Traumatol 2010;23(1):51–5.

45. Wall CR, Taylor R. Arthroscopic biceps brachii tenotomy as a treatment for canine bicipital tenosynovitis. J Am Anim Hosp Assoc 2002;38(2):169–75.

46. Cook JL, Kenter K, Fox DB. Arthroscopic biceps tenodesis: technique and results in six dogs. J Am Anim Hosp Assoc 2005;41(2):121–7.

47. Canapp SO, Canapp DA, Carr BJ, et al. Supraspinatus tendinopathy in 327 dogs: A retrospective study. VE 2016;1(3). https://doi.org/10.18849/ve.v1i3.32.

48. McDougall RA, Canapp SO, Canapp DA. Ultrasonographic Findings in 41 Dogs Treated with Bone Marrow Aspirate Concentrate and Platelet-Rich Plasma for a Supraspinatus Tendinopathy: A Retrospective Study. Front Vet Sci 2018;5:98.

49. Canapp SO, Canapp DA, Ibrahim V, et al. The Use of Adipose-Derived Progenitor Cells and Platelet-Rich Plasma Combination for the Treatment of Supraspinatus Tendinopathy in 55 Dogs: A Retrospective Study. Front Vet Sci 2016;3:61.

50. Jones SC, Howard J, Bertran J, et al. Measurement of shoulder abduction angles in dogs: an ex vivo study of accuracy and repeatability. Vet Comp Orthop Traumatol 2019;32(6):427–32.

51. von Pfeil DJF, Davis MS, Liska WD, et al. Orthopedic and ultrasonographic examination findings in 128 shoulders of 64 ultra-endurance Alaskan sled dogs. Vet Surg 2021;50(4):794–806.

52. Cook JL, Renfro DC, Tomlinson JL, et al. Measurement of angles of abduction for diagnosis of shoulder instability in dogs using goniometry and digital image analysis. Vet Surg 2005;34(5):463–8.

53. von Pfeil DJF, Megliola S, Horstman C, et al. Comparison of classic and needle arthroscopy to diagnose canine medial shoulder instability: 31 cases. Can Vet J 2021;62(5):461–8.

54. Kieves NR, Jones S. There is no superior treatment method for medial shoulder instability in dogs. VE 2020;5(1). https://doi.org/10.18849/ve.v5i1.249.

55. Nielsen C, Pluhar GE. Diagnosis and treatment of hind limb muscle strain injuries in 22 dogs. Vet Comp Orthop Traumatol 2005;18(4):247–53.

56. Cullen R, Canapp D, Dycus D, et al. Clinical Evaluation of Iliopsoas Strain with Findings from Diagnostic Musculoskeletal Ultrasound in Agility Performance Canines – 73 Cases. VE 2017;2(2). https://doi.org/10.18849/ve.v2i2.93.

57. Ragetly GR, Griffon DJ, Johnson AL, et al. Bilateral iliopsoas muscle contracture and spinous process impingement in a German Shepherd dog. Vet Surg 2009;38(8):946–53.

58. Stepnik MW, Olby N, Thompson RR, et al. Femoral neuropathy in a dog with iliopsoas muscle injury. Vet Surg 2006;35(2):186–90.

59. Hittmair KM, Groessl V, Mayrhofer E. Radiographic and ultrasonographic diagnosis of stenosing tenosynovitis of the abductor pollicis longus muscle in dogs. Vet Radiol Ultrasound 2012;53(2):135–41.

60. Entani MG, Franini A, Barella G, et al. High-Resolution Ultrasonographic Anatomy of the Carpal Tendons of Sporting Border Collies. Animals (Basel) 2022;12(16). https://doi.org/10.3390/ani12162050.

61. Tani Y. Reconstruction of the flexor carpi ulnaris tendon with a fascia lata autograft in two dogs with carpal hyperextension. Vet Surg 2022. https://doi.org/10.1111/vsu.13890.

62. Kaiser SM, Harms O, Konar M, et al. Clinical, radiographic, and magnetic resonance imaging findings of gastrocnemius musculotendinopathy in various dog breeds. Vet Comp Orthop Traumatol 2016;29(6):515–21.

63. Stahl C, Wacker C, Weber U, et al. MRI features of gastrocnemius musculotendinopathy in herding dogs. Vet Radiol Ultrasound 2010;51(4):380–5.

64. Marcellin-Little DJ, Levine D, Taylor R. Rehabilitation and conditioning of sporting dogs. Vet Clin North Am Small Anim Pract 2005;35(6):1427–39, ix.

65. Marcellin-Little DJ, Levine D, Canapp SO. The canine shoulder: selected disorders and their management with physical therapy. Clin Tech Small Anim Pract 2007;22(4):171–82.

66. Henderson AL, Latimer C, Millis DL. Rehabilitation and physical therapy for selected orthopedic conditions in veterinary patients. Vet Clin North Am Small Anim Pract 2015;45(1):91–121.

67. Brown JA, Tomlinson J. Rehabilitation of the canine forelimb. Vet Clin North Am Small Anim Pract 2021;51(2):401–20.

68. Tomlinson JE, Manfredi JM. Return to Sport after Injury: A Web-Based Survey of Owners and Handlers of Agility Dogs. Vet Comp Orthop Traumatol 2018;31(6):473–8.

69. Heidorn SN, Canapp SO Jr, Zink CM, et al. Rate of return to agility competition for dogs with cranial cruciate ligament tears treated with tibial plateau leveling osteotomy. J Am Vet Med Assoc 2018;253(11):1439–44.

70. Kieves NR, Shoben AB, Pechette Markley A. Treatment and Outcome of Thoracic and Pelvic Limb Injuries Sustained By Agility Dogs. 21st ESVOT Congress Proc 2022.

71.. Inkilä L, Hyytiäinen HK, Hielm-Björkman A, et al. Part I of Finnish Agility Dog Survey: Training and Management of Competition-Level Agility Dogs. Animals (Basel) 2022;12(2):212.

Rehabilitation Therapy for the Degenerative Myelopathy Patient

Theresa E. Pancotto, DVM, MS, CCRP

KEYWORDS

- Degenerative myelopathy • Dog • Physical rehabilitation • Neurology

KEY POINTS

- Physical rehabilitation exercises, both active and passive, have been demonstrated to improve survival times in dogs diagnosed with degenerative myelopathy.
- Therapeutic modalities such as acupuncture, photobiomodulation, and electrical stimulation may help some patients, but robust data are lacking.
- Regular functional and qualitative assessments are helpful in making decisions for patients with degenerative myelopathy.

INTRODUCTION

Degenerative myelopathy (DM) is a progressive, neurodegenerative disease caused by an inherited mutation in the SOD-1 gene. The clinical condition was first reported in 1973 by Averill[1] and the underlying cause was later determined by Awano and colleagues in 2009.[2] Although the condition is genetic and most affected dogs are homozygous for the mutation, penetrance is incomplete.[3] The most common breeds affected with the SOD1:c.118 A mutation include German Shepherds, Pembroke Welsh Corgi, Boxer, Rhodesian Ridgeback, and Chesapeake Bay Retriever.[4] Although the exact mechanism of neurodegeneration is unclear, accumulations of misfolded SOD1 proteins and toxic gain of function have been reported [2,5]

EVALUATION

Initial clinical signs are consistent with asymmetric, non-painful T3–L3 myelopathy.[1] In my experience, dogs with DM maintain an intact cutaneous trunci reflex, though this finding has not been explored definitively. There is no sex predilection and most dogs are at least 8 years old at the onset of clinical signs.[1,6–12] Loss of myotactic and withdrawal reflexes in the pelvic limbs occur in later stages of the disease[1,6,8,10,12] and peripheral nerves may be involved.[2] Although survival may exceed 3 years, humane

2575 Northbrooke Plaza Drive, Building 100, Naples, FL 34119, USA
E-mail address: tep0008@auburn.edu

Vet Clin Small Anim 53 (2023) 845–856
https://doi.org/10.1016/j.cvsm.2023.02.017
0195-5616/23/Published by Elsevier Inc.
vetsmall.theclinics.com

euthanasia is frequently elected when the disease has progressed to paraplegia. Over time, the disease will progress to involve thoracic limbs and eventually respiratory centers. The involvement of medullary respiratory centers is associated with death.[5] Corgis have been shown to survive longer, though it is unknown if they have a unique form of the disease or if they are more manageable due to their smaller size.[11]

Although definitive diagnosis can only be established histopathologically,[13] the clinician has access to numerous tests to help support or refute the likelihood of DM as an etiologic diagnosis. Genetic testing is now readily available through the Orthopedic Foundation for Animals (ofa.org) and other at-home DNA test kits. One must be cautious as to the quality of testing provided, because improperly designed DNA amplification primers may lead to misdiagnosis.[14] As stated above, SOD1:c.118 A/A homozygotes are most likely to be affected, though some dogs may never develop clinical DM due to incomplete penetrance. Heterozygotes (SOD1:c.118 A/G) are considered at risk and wild-type (SOD1:c.118 G/G) is least at risk though there are scarce reports of wild-type animals with histopathologically confirmed DM.[4] Additionally, the Bernese Mountain dog affected by DM suffers from an alternate mutation in the same gene SOD1:c52 T.[15]

Routine MRI is helpful for ruling out structural causes that may look clinically similar such as chronic or type II intervertebral disk disease and slow-growing neoplasia. It is possible for a patient to have more than one disease contributing to the clinical picture and these patients may present both diagnostic and therapeutic challenges. Cerebrospinal fluid (CSF) analysis has some changes seen with DM but is not specific to that disease.[13] Among the changes reported include elevated myelin basic protein, increased oligoclonal bands, and increased phosphorylated neurofilament heavy chain protein (pNFh).[3,13] Increased CSF PNFh has shown some promise in being able to differentiate dogs with DM versus other chronic, progressive neurologic conditions.[3]

Diffusion tensor imaging (DTI) enables in vivo quantification of the movement of water molecules and can provide useful information on spinal cord integrity. Both decreased ADC (apparent diffusion coefficient) and FA (fractional anisotropy) values have been identified in dogs with DM.[16,17] The suspected decrease in ADC and FA is attributed to axonal damage and the change in water content due to cytotoxic edema as well as the change in lipid due to demyelination.[16] These studies are promising, and DTI will be immensely helpful in characterizing DM at the time of clinical onset. Unfortunately, the exact parameters, sensitivity, and specificity remain to be determined.

Steroid-response trials have been anecdotally reported as a therapeutic trial for non-DM cases but may yield a false-positive steroid "boost" or non-specific treatment response due to anti-inflammatory effects on comorbidities (eg, osteoarthritis, chronic disk disease) in dogs with DM.

CURRENT EVIDENCE FOR PHYSICAL REHABILITATION AND COMPLEMENTARY MEDICINE

There is no cure for DM, however, physical rehabilitation (PR) has shown improved survival times with sustained periods of ambulation. Kathmann and colleagues[18] demonstrated that dogs undergoing moderate PR lived an average of 130 days versus 55 days with no PR. Dogs undergoing intensive PR lived an average of 255 days. Both groups receiving PR showed statistically significantly longer survival times than those who did not.[18]

The progression of DM is gradual, even in the face of PR. It has been my experience that dogs undergoing PR will decline in a stair-step fashion, rather than steadily over time. Most dogs will plateau for a period and then have a sudden decline, followed by another plateau, and so on.

Any PR program should consist of paw protection, active exercises, passive exercises, massage, and hydrotherapy, if possible.[19] The latter is the most technical and equipment-intensive component. Unfortunately, no studies have evaluated the individual effects of therapies within these categories (**Table 1**).

Paw protection can be achieved using a variety of products from baby socks to heavy-duty canine shoes. Many products made especially for handicapped dogs now exist and can be purchased online or at local pet retail stores. Initially, patients only need light coverage to avoid wearing of the digits and bleeding at the nail bed (**Fig. 1**A–C). As weakness increases, sturdier protection is warranted (**Fig. 2**). Although this can provide some resistance to work against, it may also contribute to increased dragging from the sheer weight of the shoe. Toe-up devices are shoe alternatives that minimize dragging without being excessively heavy (**Fig. 3**). These devices have the added benefit of breathability for the feet and can be used on an underwater treadmill. Cuttable resistance bands can be looped around the metatarsals and either tied to a harness or manually pulled forward. Trial and error with the weight and length of the band is needed to ensure a proper fit and appropriate resistance/support.

Active exercises encourage maximum voluntary muscle recruitment to maintain strength. The most basic active exercise is walking over a flat surface. Early in the course of the disease, this can be made more difficult by walking uphill, through sand, across a mattress, or over obstacles (cavaletti rails). Sit-to-stand exercises are another easy and often already-known exercise for many patients. Difficulty can be increased by adding a weighted vest or decreased by providing assistance with a sling or harness or reducing the range of motion by having the patient sit on an elevated surface. Weight shifting on a variety of surfaces (flat ground, physio disk, mattress, wobble board) improves and maintains balance. As with any PR program, exercises should be adapted to the patient's motivation and physical condition, providing more support to the patient as the disease progresses. In general, short, frequent periods of exercise are preferred to long, sustained periods.[18] Current recommendations are for 5 to 10 minutes at least five times per day.[18]

Transcutaneous electrical stimulation is an alternative way to elicit muscle contraction. Electrically stimulated muscle contractions are always less strong than voluntary contractions; they are usually not indicated unless patients have minimal to no motor function. This type of stimulation may be uncomfortable to some patients. No studies have evaluated the effects of transcutaneous electrical stimulation on outcomes in dogs with DM.

Passive exercises are performed primarily to maintain joint and muscle health, but do not build muscle. Passive range of motion should be performed at each joint, starting distally and moving proximally. The movements should be slow and gentle through both flexion and extension within the patient's comfortable and physiologic range of motion. Massage is another passive exercise performed to ease muscle pain and improve blood flow. Massage of the pelvic limbs is important for blood and lymphatic flow, particularly in non-ambulatory patients. Thoracic and epaxial massage may be more focused on identifying tight areas associated with compensation and front-loading of body weight secondary to chronic weakness. The iliopsoas is a muscle prone to tightness and may be exquisitely sensitive to massage. Topical heat or therapeutic ultrasound may be beneficial in relaxing this muscle before massage. Reverse brushing, or brushing against the fur growth, may help improve proprioception and body awareness without asking anything from the patient. Although this might be irritating for dogs who have minimal dysfunction, it may be enjoyable to those who

Table 1
Rehabilitation exercise recommendations from Kathmann et al[18]

	Instruction	Duration and Frequency
Active Exercise	• Slow walking • If needed, knuckling is prevented by a sling around the paw and pulling the dog's limb by each step with it • Frequent exercises preferred to long exercise • Exercise has to be adapted to animal's condition • Dog sits and gets up several times • Assistance with sling if needed • Attention is paid to correct placement of the paws • Weight shifting while standing: making the dog bear his weight once on the left, then on the right side by pushing him gently at the level of the hip • Changing of ground (grass, asphalt, sand) • Stair climbing, walking uphill	5–10 min at least 5 times/d
Passive exercise	• Gentle, slow extension and flexion of each joint of both hind limbs (starting distally, manipulating of each joint performed separately) • Maintaining the range of physiologic motion of each joint • The limb is always fixed proximally to the joint and the distal part is moved	3 times/d, 10 times in each articulation
Massage	• Massage is started and finished with stroking • Gentle massage (kneading) of the entire paravertebral muscles and the limbs, starting from distal to proximal	3 times/d
Hydrotherapy	• If available, walking on underwater treadmill; otherwise, swimming or walking in water, depending on dog's ability • Adaptation to animal's condition is important • Assistance with a sling as needed • Weight shifting while standing in water: making the dog bear it's weight once on the left, then on the right by pushing him gently at the level of the hip	At least once a week, 5–20 min
Paw protection	• With a bandage or socks and shoes	While walking

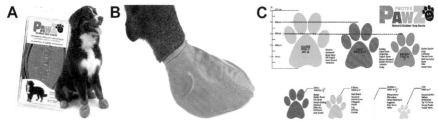

Fig. 1. (*A*) Light foot protection. X-large rubber dog boot. Photo courtesy of Pawz Dog Boots. Tip for outdoor use: When your dog drags his paw, there is probably one spot that will get worn quicker due to the friction. To help reinforce and extend the longevity of the boot, you can place a piece of duct tape or gorilla glue over the sweet spot. Also, the boot does not have a specific top or bottom. You do not need to cover the dew claw. Some customers place a baby sock under the boot for extra cushioning. If you are placing the boot over a bandage, we recommend that you go up a full size to accommodate the wrap. Tip for indoor use: Because the boots are waterproof (great for keeping the elements out), the boots do not breathe. The boots have the same properties that a swim cap would have. To help make the boot less constricting for indoor use, carefully cut the roll off the top of the boot. The boot will stay on. Use a single-hole punch to actually punch holes in the boots so any moisture that should build up will evaporate. Please make sure to monitor your pet and to remove the boots frequently to make sure your pooch is comfortable. Each dog has their tolerance level so it will be important to find your dog's threshold. (*B*) Light foot protection. Close-up of large dog boot. Link for how to put boots on: https://vimeo.com/81364925. (*C*) Pawz size chart (PDF). (Photo courtesy of Pawz Dog Boots.)

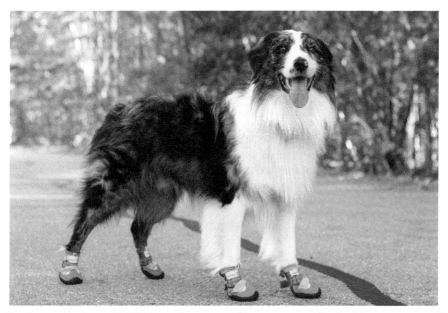

Fig. 2. Durable boot. Walkin'Boots feature a rubber, waterproof sole. (Photo courtesy of Walkin'Pets.)

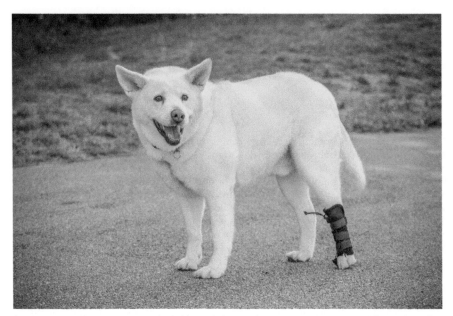

Fig. 3. Toe-up device. Rear no-knuckle training sock encourages pets to pick up their feet when knuckling or dragging their rear paws. (Photo courtesy of Walkin'Pets).

spend longer periods in recumbency. These hands-on, full-body interventions are good opportunities to look for decubital ulcers or wounds associated with increasing weakness and recumbency. Current recommendations for joint range of motion and body massage are for three times per day; 10 reps at each joint[18] and 5 to 10 minutes of massage.

Hydrotherapy includes both swimming and walking in water. If using a natural water source for walking, one should evaluate the floor to avoid particularly sharp or slippery surfaces. Underwater treadmills are preferred for the control of the environment and speed of walking. Walking in water establishes a more normal gait pattern than is achieved with swimming,[20] though swimming is still a good option if an underwater treadmill is not available. Many non-water-loving dogs will accept the underwater treadmill because water rises slowly from the bottom rather than immediate submersion or coming from the top like a bathtub.[20] Lifejackets are recommended in general but additional buoyancy for the pelvic limbs in weak dogs may be provided with a support harness, foam noodles, or other inflatable devices that can be adjusted to the patient's body size. Flotation devices that fit under the belly are good for support but may discourage pelvic limb movement due to constant contact of the hip flexors. If you are working in a pool, the owner/handler/trainer can provide manual support by lifting the back end from underneath the pelvis or by using a support harness. Current recommendations for hydrotherapy are for a minimum of one session per week, 5 to 20 minutes.[18]

There is little research on using specific modalities in patients with DM. Miller and colleagues[21] retrospectively compared two photobiomodulation (PBMt) protocols in addition to a standardized PR protocol in patients suspected to have DM.

Protocol-A[21]: Protocol-B[21]:
Wavelength 904 nm 980 nm.
Radiant power 0.5 W 6 to 12 W.

Irradiance at skin 0.5 W/cm^2 1.2 to 2.4 W/cm^2.

Fluence 8 J/cm^2, per point 14 to 21, average over treatment area.

Point-to-point grid method, 20 points continuously moving grid.

Treatment area 650 to 1000 cm^2 650 to 1000 cm^2.

Treatment time 5 min 20 sec 25 to 26 min, 15 sec.

Diagnostic criteria for each patient were variable and ranged from genetic testing and clinical signs to post-mortem histopathological evidence. Dogs in Protocol-B had a statistically significantly longer time between onset of signs and non-ambulatory paresis as well as between onset of signs and euthanasia.[21] Importantly, dogs in Protocol-B also had statistically significantly longer time of onset of clinical symptoms to start of treatment, which suggests that they may have had an overall less severe form of the disease. Additionally, there are concerns over the possibility of laser therapy worsening the disease state. The mutation that causes DM is a toxic *gain of function* mutation, which leads to an excess in anti-oxidant activity, thereby, damaging the neural tissue.[2,5] As a stimulatory treatment, the potential for the laser to further increase anti-oxidant function exists and its application to the spinal cord should be considered with caution. Conversely, new data have demonstrated micro-inflammation in the spinal cords of dogs diagnosed with DM[22] and it is possible that certain laser treatment protocols may modify the microenvironment, reduce inflammation, and slow disease progression. The benefit of photobiomodulation may also be related to non-neural stimulation, improving blood flow to muscles, reducing oxidative stress, and preventing exercise-induced fatigue.[21]

Curcumin was associated with statistically longer survival times (43 vs 34 months) in a study that monitored Pembroke Welsh Corgis with DM from diagnosis to natural death.[5] Curcumin molecules have been shown to bind to the aggregation-prone regions of the mutant SOD1 protein and block the formation of unstructured aggregates.[23] There are also documented benefits in muscle leading to increased protein synthesis, reduced protein degradation, and fewer exercise-induced muscle injuries.[24,25] The curcumin dose was 13 mg given orally once per day or divided and given twice per day. Unfortunately, this study did not control for other complementary treatments or PR and the authors consented that survival effects may have been due to a combination of treatments and the client's general approach to care rather than to curcumin specifically.[5]

Acupuncture for analgesia is growing in veterinary medicine. Although a complete review of the mechanisms and benefits of acupuncture is beyond the scope of this article, the reader is urged to consider incorporating acupuncture in the management of dogs with DM. Traditional acupuncture as well as dry-needling of trigger points can offer therapeutic advantages by providing non-pharmaceutical ways to address pain in muscles and joints that may be over-taxed by chronic off-loading or those which are affected by comorbid diseases such as osteoarthritis.[26]

In animal models and in older people suffering from stroke, combined rehabilitation and acupuncture proved superior results in cognitive function as well as motor function compared with those with physical exercise alone.[27,28] Spinal cord injury models in rats have shown promising results on axonal regeneration with the application of electroacupuncture after spinal cord injury.[29] The application of such novel work still needs to be applied to canine degenerative spinal cord disease.

Patients who have progressed to paraplegia are no longer able to participate in active exercises that engage the pelvic limbs and they may lack motivation on some days. Daily physical movement is still important and can be aided by use of a supportive harness (**Figs. 4** and **5**), sling, wheelchair, or cart (**Figs. 6** and **7**). These patients continue to benefit from massage, passive range of motion, acupuncture,

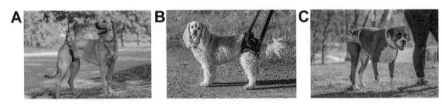

Fig. 4. Rear limb harness. (*A*) Minimal contact Walkin' Up-n-Go leash. Great for male dogs or those who are inhibited by thicker fabrics with more body contact. (*B*) Neoprene rear lift harness by Walkin'Pets. (*C*) Warrior sling by Walkin'Pets that can be used with or without a wheelchair for easy transitions. (Photo courtesy of Walkin'Pets.)

and heat. Utilizing an UWTM or heated pool with jets can also be therapeutic by easing joint and muscle pain and providing some whole-body sensory stimulus. I think of these complementary-therapy-intense days as "spa days" where I ask very little of the patient and focus on making them comfortable.

CLINICAL OUTCOMES

Objective data can be helpful in making important life decisions. There are several good objective scoring systems that can be applied to patients with DM. It is important to have a client fill out an assessment form at the beginning as a baseline and every 1 to 3 months for monitoring. Because it is necessary to adapt one's lifestyle as DM patients deteriorate, it can be hard to maintain objectivity on what a good quality of life is. The objective scoring systems can help maintain integrity in our value systems and provide perspective on the situation.

Although DM is a non-painful condition, pain may develop over time as other muscles compensate for weakness and/or if complications arise from using various assistive devices or having long recumbent periods. Device modification such as strategically placed extra padding can be helpful. The Canine Brief Pain Inventory[30] may be a helpful assessment tool for some of these patients but could need modifications or be used as one of several assessment tools. The Hurt, Hunger, Hydration, Hygiene, Happiness, Mobility, and More-good-days-than-bad Scale (HHHHHMM Scale) is a concept developed by Dr Alice Villalobos and has been adopted and adapted by different institutions to create quality-of-life surveys that help guide clients with terminal decisions.[31] When asking a client to fill these out shortly after diagnosis, it is important to remind them that it is simply a baseline measurement and does not imply that euthanasia is in the near future.

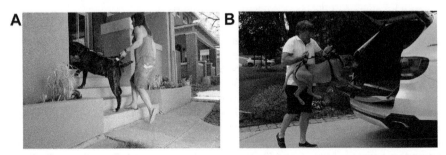

Fig. 5. Full body harness. (*A*) Help'em Up full body support with rear limb assistance (*B*) Help'em Up full body harness with full assist. (Photo courtesy of Paw Prosper.)

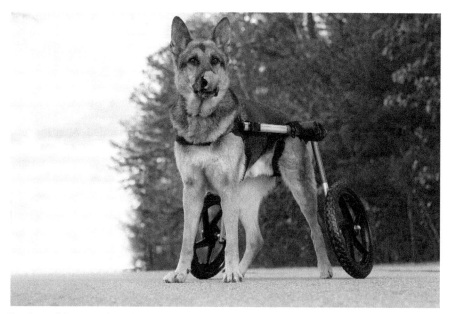

Fig. 6. Walkin'Pets wheelchair. Adjustable wheelchair with customizable frames and colored wheels. (Photo courtesy of Walkin'Pets.)

CLIENT COMMUNICATION

It is important to spend time with the client not only explaining the disease and progression, but to demonstrate appropriate PR techniques. Although the Kathmann[18] prescription includes approximately six specific exercises adapted to individual patient function and motivation, this may be an overwhelming place for a client to begin. I advocate for starting with just two to three recommended at-home exercises and I add one exercise every 1 to 2 weeks if compliance is good. I request that clients video-record themselves performing exercises at home so I can ensure appropriate

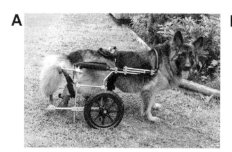
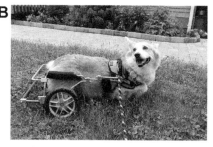

Fig. 7. Counter balance wheelchair. (*A*) The German shepherd's cart is in the fully counterbalanced position, feet are in stirrups, wheels forward and yoke weightless on the shoulders, so the axle is relieving up to 35% of the weight borne on the forelimbs. (*B*) The corgi's cart is set at a slight counterbalance, with the weight of her rump behind the wheels relieving a percentage of weight normally carried on the front legs. You can see the variable axle in this photo—as you locate the wheels forward, a greater percentage of weight is lifted off the forelimbs, giving DM dogs a longer period of independence and mobility as the disease progresses. (Photo courtesy of Eddie's Wheels).

technique and create modifications, if needed, based on lifestyle, environment, and available assistance.

A strong argument can be made for at-home euthanasia for these patients. They generally are not so sick that the facilities of a veterinary hospital are required. However, these are also patients who have frequented the hospital for their weekly PR and may not have the typical negative associations of many sick patients. Either way, we want to prioritize a comfortable environment for saying goodbye. Best practices for euthanasia such as oral or injectable pre-medications as advocated for by the Companion Animal Euthanasia Training Academy should be implemented. After the time and dedication many clients give to their dogs with DM, grief counseling may help many clients through this journey successfully.

DISCUSSION

Although there is evidence to support the use of physical exercise in slowing progression of DM, there remain a great many unknowns about specific applications of isolated exercises and individual therapeutic modalities. Future studies are needed specifically investigating the application of treatments such as laser therapy, electrical stimulation, and acupuncture including the parameters for treatment, frequency of application, and clinical and neurophysiological outcomes.

SUMMARY

Clinicians should encourage their clients to pursue appropriate testing for an accurate diagnosis of DM. Advanced imaging with MRI and a positive genetic test are the current standards of care for obtaining an appropriate diagnosis. Although a diagnosis of multi-focal type II disk disease may not change your therapeutic plan, it will inform both you and the client of expected progression. Physical exercise and a variety of therapeutic modalities should be applied to maximize results but use caution when safety has not been demonstrated. Lastly, use a variety of client surveys to gauge the quality of life and provide perspective when dealing with a terminal illness.

CLINICS CARE POINTS

- Accurate diagnostic testing provides useful information regarding underlying disease(s), prognosis and comorbidities.
- Variety of physical rehabilitation exercises including different passive and active exercises is paramount in designing a patient program. Be adaptable and indulge on some days when motivation may be low.
- Use client surveys to help track the quality of life and provide perspective on patient progression.

DISCLOSURE

Nothing to disclose.

REFERENCES

1. Averill DR. Degenerative myelopathy in the aging German shepherd dog: clinical and pathologic findings. J Am Vet Med Assoc 1973;162(12):1045–51.

2. Awano T, Johnson GS, Wade CM, et al. Genome-wide association analysis reveals a SOD1 mutation in canine degenerative myelopathy that resembles amyotrophic lateral sclerosis. Proc Natl Acad Sci USA 2009;106(8):2794–9.

3. Toedebusch CM, Bachrach MD, Garcia VB, et al. Cerebrospinal fluid levels of phosphorylated neurofilament heavy as a diagnostic marker of canine degenerative myelopathy. J Vet Intern Med 2017;31:502–13.

4. Zeng R, Coates JR, Johnson GC, et al. Breed distribution of SOD1 alleles previously associated with canine degenerative myelopathy. J Vet Int Med 2014;28:515–21.

5. Kobatake Y, Nakata K, Sakai H, et al. The long-term clinical course of canine degenerative myelopathy and therapeutic potential of curcumin. Veterinary Sciences 2021;8:192.

6. Griffiths IR, Duncan ID. Chronic degenerative radiculomyelopathy in the dog. J Sm Anim Pract 1975;16:461–71.

7. Braund KG, Vandevelde M. German shepherd dog myelopathy – a morphologic and morphometric study. Am J Vet Res 1978;39:1309–15.

8. Coates JR, March PA, Oglesbee M, et al. Clinical characterization of a familial degenerative myelopathy in Pembroke Welsh corgi dogs. J Vet Intern Med 2007;21:1323–31.

9. Johnston PE, Barrie JA, McCulloch MC, et al. Central nervous system pathology in 25 dogs with chronic degenerative radiculomyelopathy. Vet Rec 2000;146:629–33.

10. Matthews NS, de Lahunta A. Degenerative myelopathy in an adult miniature poodle. J Am Vet Med Assoc 1985;186:1213–5.

11. March P, Coates JR, Abyad RJ, et al. Degenerative myelopathy in 18 Pembroke Welsh corgi dogs. Vet Pathol 2009;46(2):241–50.

12. Bischsel P, Vandevelde M, Lang J, et al. Degenerative myelopathy in a family of Siberian husky dogs. J Am Vet Med Assoc 1983;183:998–1000.

13. Coates JR, Wininger FA. Canine Degenerative Myelopathy. Vet Clin Small Anim 2010;40:929–50.

14. Turba ME, Loechel R, Rombola E, et al. Evidence of a genomic insertion in intron 2 of SOD1 causing allelic drop-out during routine diagnostic testing for canine degenerative myelopathy. Anim Genet 2016;48:365–8.

15. Wininger FA, Zeng R, Johnson GS, et al. Degenerative myelopathy in a Bernese mountain dog with a novel SOD1 missense mutation. J Vet Intern Med 2011;25(5):1166–70.

16. Naito E, Nakata K, Sakai H, et al. Diffusion tensor imaging-based quantitative analysis of the spinal cord in Pembroke Welsh corgis with degenerative myelopathy. J Vet Med Sci 2022;84(2):199–207.

17. Johnson PF, Miller AD, Cheetham J, et al. In vivo detection of microstructural spinal cord lesions in dogs with degenerative myelopathy using diffusion tensor imaging. J Vet Intern Med 2021;35:352–62.

18. Kahmann I, Cizinauskas S, Doherr MG, et al. Daily controlled physiotherapy increases survival time in dogs with suspected degenerative myelopathy. J Vet Intern Med 2006;20(4):927–32.

19. Spinella G, Bettella P, Riccio B, et al. Overview of the current literature on the most common neurological diseases in dogs with a particular focus on rehabilitation. Veterinary Sciences 2022;9:429.

20. Millis DL, Levine D. Canine rehabilitation and physical therapy. 2nd edition. Saunders (Elsevier); 2013.

21. Miller LA, Torraca DG, De Taboada L. Retrospective observational study and analysis of two different photobiomodulation therapy protocols combined with rehabilitation therapy as therapeutic interventions for canine degenerative myelopathy. Photobiomodulation, Photomedicine, and Laser Surgery 2020; 38(4):195–205.
22. Hashimoto K, Kobatake Y, Asahina R, et al. Up-regulated inflammatory signatures of the spinal cord in canine degenerative myelopathy. Res Vet Sci 2021;135: 442–9.
23. Bhatia NK, Srivastava A, Katyal N, et al. Curcumin binds to the pre-fibrillar aggregates of Cu/Zn superoxide dismutase (SOD1) and alters its amyloidogenic pathway resulting in reduced cytotoxicity. Biochim Biophys Acta 2015;1854: 426–36.
24. Fang W, Nasi Y. The effect of curcumin supplementation on recovery following exercise-induced muscle damage and delayed-onset muscle soreness: a systematic review and meta-analysis of randomized controlled trials. Phytother Res 2021;35:1768–81.
25. Manas-Garcia L, Bargall N, Gea J, et al. Muscle phenotype, proteolysis, and atrophy signaling during reloading in mice: effects of curcumin on the gastrocnemius. Nutrients 2020;12:388.
26. Fry LM, Neary SM, Sharrock J, et al. Acupuncture for analgesia in veterinary medicine. Top Companion Anim Med 2014;29(2):35–42.
27. Zhang P, Jiang G, Wang Q, et al. Effects of early acupuncture combined with rehabilitation training on limb function and nerve injury rehabilitation in elderly patients with stroke: based on a retrospective cohort study. BioMed Res Int 2022;23.
28. Wang D, Li L, Zhang Q, et al. Combination of electroacupuncture and constraint-induced movement therapy enhances functional recovery after ischemic stroke in rats. J Mol Neurosci 2021;71(10):2116–25.
29. Tan C, Yang C, Liu H, et al. Effect of Schwann cell transplantation combined with electroacupuncture on axonal regeneration and remyelination in raths with spinal cord injury. Anat Rec 2021;304(11):2506–20.
30. Brown D, Boston R, Coyne J, et al. A novel approach to the use of animals in studies of pain: development of the canine brief pain inventory (CBPI). J Pain 2007;8(4):S5.
31. Villalobos A, Kaplan L. Canine and Feline Geriatric Oncology: honoring the human-animal bond. Blackwell Publishing; 2007. p. 370.

Therapy Exercises Following Cranial Cruciate Ligament Repair in Dogs

Molly J. Flaherty, DVM, CCRP, CVA, CVSMT, CVPP

KEYWORDS

- Therapeutic exercise • Postoperative rehabilitation • Cranial cruciate ligament
- Veterinary orthopedic • Canine rehabilitation

KEY POINTS

- Land-based exercises using minimal equipment can be used to maximize functional outcome following cranial cruciate ligament repair in dogs.
- Exercises can be demonstrated to pet owners for at home therapy.
- Research evidence supports benefits for dogs receiving rehabilitation therapy following cruciate ligament repair surgery.
- Goals of therapy exercises include improved joint range of motion, proprioception, weight-bearing, muscle mass, strength, balance, and prevention of injury.

 Video content accompanies this article at http://www.vetsmall.theclinics.com.

INTRODUCTION

Rehabilitation therapy for postsurgical orthopedic veterinary patients has gained awareness for its benefits including improving range of motion, posture, proprioception, muscle mass, gait retraining, strengthening, and endurance. Rehabilitation therapy has been regarded as necessary for the recovery of correct functionality of the limb in a review of the biomechanics and etiopathogenetic factors concerning cranial cruciate rupture in dogs.[1] Surgery for cranial cruciate ligament (CCL) repair is one of the most common orthopedic procedures in dogs. Supporting evidence exists for benefits of rehabilitation in postoperative CLL surgery patients.[2–4] After tibial plateau leveling osteotomy (TPLO) procedure, physiotherapy can enhance muscle mass and strength, stifle range of motion and prevention of muscle atrophy.[4] Rehabilitation therapy in early limb use has been suggested to improve range of motion, muscle mass and strength, balance, reduce lameness, and help prevent further injury.[5] A survey

Department of Clinical Sciences, Ryan Veterinary Hospital, School of Veterinary Medicine, University of Pennsylvania, 3900 Delancey St., Philadelphia, PA 19104, USA
E-mail address: Mollyfl@vet.upenn.edu

Vet Clin Small Anim 53 (2023) 857–868
https://doi.org/10.1016/j.cvsm.2023.02.013
0195-5616/23/© 2023 Elsevier Inc. All rights reserved.

of veterinarians performing surgical treatment of CCL disease found a high proportion recommend postoperative rehabilitation therapy.[6]

Clients may not have access to these benefits because of lack of local rehabilitation facilities or financial limitations. These patients are generally in veterinary contact during the initial 8-week recovery period and then may be lost to follow-up. The early postoperative period is the optimal time when therapy can improve outcome and veterinary-patient contact is present.

The goals of this article are to review postoperative CCL rehabilitation therapy for dogs during the first 8 weeks postoperative. The exercises reviewed are those which can be done with minimal equipment such as balance discs, cushions, cavaletti rails, stairs and low incline hills, making it easy to incorporate in home care. The exercises described in this article should first be demonstrated in the clinic for client education. These exercises are practical for most CCL surgeries such as TPLO, tibial tuberosity advancement, and extracapsular techniques. Nonsurgical or medical management cases of CCL injury can also follow a similar protocol but the initial rest and inflammatory reduction phase may need to be prolonged an additional week or more. In the case of nonsurgical medical management, it should be kept in mind that there may be instability and exercises that cause discomfort should be discontinued.

When possible, a full service rehabilitation facility should be recommended because they can provide guidance, more options, and a tailored program. In cases where additional surgery was done, such as patella luxation correction, care should be noted on exercises that may cause stretch of the patella tendon early on, such as sit to stand exercise. This exercise may be delayed an additional week or more. Communication with the orthopedic surgeon is essential to be aware of any changes or concerns for each patient.

Programs for home exercise should be kept simple to not overwhelm pet owners, improve compliance, and reduce risks of complications. Suggested frequency is daily the first 2 weeks and 4 to 6 days per week for 15 to 20 minutes of time weeks 3 to 8. Weaker animals may require a reduced duration of time and repetitions. When patients have limited physical capability, even simple techniques such as massage, range of motion, and isometric standing exercises can be recommended that will have an influence on improving recovery. The physical ability of the pet owner should also be a consideration when choosing home exercises to ensure the ability to carry through.

THE FIRST 72 HOURS

During the acute inflammatory phase of recovery, which is generally the first 72 hours, treatments may be done in the hospital and continued at home for those discharged. This time period is focused on reducing inflammation, pain control, beginning range of motion and stimulation of vascularization and healing.[7] Therapy may include cryotherapy, passive range of motion (PROM), massage, weight shifting and supported walking.

Cryotherapy is known to produce vasoconstriction; decreasing local blood flow, inflammatory response and edema, thereby reducing pain. Skin and underlying tissue temperatures can be decreased to a depth of 2 to 4 cm, decreasing conduction velocity of pain nerve signals.[8] Cold therapy using gel-filled or grain-filled ice packs can be applied 2 to 4 times daily for 10 to 20 minutes for the first 3 to 5 days after surgery.

PROM is a technique that allows for the diffusion of nutrients from synovial fluid to cartilage, improves circulation and flexibility, and reduces tension of periarticular muscles. The technique involves moving all limb joints through their range of flexion and extension in a sagittal plane, working with each joint individually from distal to proximal. Patients should be laying in lateral recumbency and calm. Surgical joints can be painful and have limited range of motion that will require slow, careful motion to apply PROM safely. The limb should be supported above and below the joint and then place the joint slowly into flexion and then into extension. This should only be done to a degree that does not cause pain or tissue trauma and is not pushed beyond what feels natural (Video 1). End range of motion will be more limited in the acute postoperative joint due to inflammation and swelling. Treatments should comprise 10 to 15 repetitions every 6 to 8 hours.

Massage aids in myofascial release, enhances circulation, reduces edema, minimizes muscle contraction and scarring, and reduces painful muscle spasms. Techniques commonly used for animal patients are stroking, effleurage, and petrissage. Stroking is slow gliding movements over the body using the palm of the hand in the direction of fur growth, cranial to caudal, and proximal to distal. This helps in relaxation and increase blood flow to the areas applied. Effleurage helps with fluid mobilization and lymphatic drainage; the palms of the whole hand are used for long strokes with light-to-moderate pressure distal to proximal and along the direction of muscle fibers toward the flow of lymphatic and drainage back to the heart. Petrissage uses kneading, compression, tissue squeezing, and skin rolling with moderate pressure. This technique helps restore tissue mobility and assist with lymphatic return. It is important to assure that massage is not uncomfortable to the patient and not used over areas of tissue trauma such as directly over a healing surgical area. Areas commonly focused on after hind limb surgery are the shoulders and hip flexors. These are areas that often take on compensatory muscle tension due to altered weight-bearing distribution and gait patterns.

Therapy exercises during this time period should be limited to standing weight shifting and supported walking. Slings or harnesses can be used to help support the patient. Flooring should have good footing and covered with yoga mats or traction mats if the surface is slick. Patients are usually non–weight-bearing to toe touching at this phase. Standing weight shifting should be gentle and limited to causing mild unbalance to elicit toe touching to the floor. This can be done for 1 minute 3 to 4 times per day. Supported walking should be slow and controlled is limited to short time periods of less than 5 minutes to eliminate.

FIRST 72 HOURS TO 2 WEEKS

Patients are generally in home recovery and clients will need direction for therapy. This time period is focused on improving the range of motion, isometric weight-bearing and reducing compensatory problems in other muscle areas. PROM should be continued and cryotherapy as needed. Slow leash walks to eliminate are generally still limited to 5 minutes, 3 to 4 times per day. Exercises commonly introduced to patients at this time include weight shifting on a soft foam pad and stretches. During this phase of recovery, stress on the patellar tendon should be avoided to prevent patellar tendinopathy. Excessive flexion during weight-bearing is avoided and activities such as jumping, running, stairs, and crouched walking position are not advised.[9]

Weight shifting exercises can be started on the ground level if the patient has minimal to no weight-bearing on the surgical limb. For animals that are already bearing some weight, the challenge can be increased by having their front paws or all 4 limbs on a low-balance pad or cushion (**Fig. 1**). Their body weight is shifted with gentle nudges to elicit limb lowering and weight placement onto the affected limb. Movements should be gentle enough to not cause stumbling but to obtain the desired effect. For some animals, this exercise will work better by directing head motion up

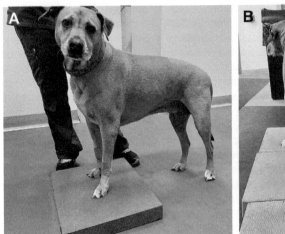
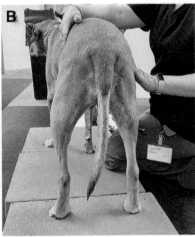

Fig. 1. Weight shifting (*A*) Forelimbs on balance pad (*B*) All 4 limbs on balance pads.

and down and side to side in response for a food reward or toy. The head movements will cause mild weight shifting and can be directed for a specific limb. For example, head motion upward will shift weight to the hind limbs and to the right will shift more weight to the right side. Weight shifting can be done for 30 to 60 seconds for 1 to 3 repetitions.

Stretching can help to reduce compensatory problems including muscle tension in areas of the body taking extraload during recovery. Some stretches will also help in improving weight-bearing onto the desired limb. Two stretches that patients can often do during this phase of recovery are side bends and low step-up stretches. Side bends are also commonly referred to as cookie stretches. Because the pet is standing, the head is guiding to the right and then to left shoulder region in response to a food reward or toy. The head should be held for 5 to 10 seconds in the right and left position. The stretch can be taken first to shoulder then chest; if the patient is able to maintain form and balance, the stretch can then be continued to the hip (**Fig. 2**). This exercise will stretch through the neck and shoulders, which are common areas of tension following hind limb lameness. Because the head turns to the right and left, mild weight shifting is also elicited to the hind limbs on the same side, and paraspinal and cervical muscles are stretched on the opposite side.

Step-up stretch involves having the patient place their front limbs up on a low elevation (**Fig. 3**). The height of forelimb elevation will be dependent on the size of the animal and their comfort in hip extension. This exercise will aid in increasing weight-bearing to

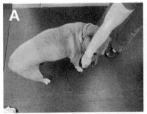
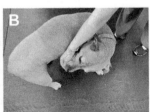
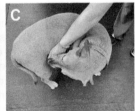

Fig. 2. Side bend stretches (*A*) to shoulder level (*B*) to chest level (*C*) to hip level.

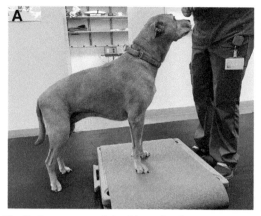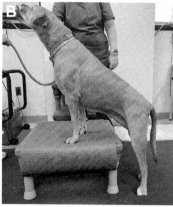

Fig. 3. Step-up stretch for hip and stifle extension. (*A*) The step can be set lower for patients unable to fully extend their joints comfortably (*B*) At a higher level for more hip extension.

the hind limbs and in improving hip extension. Following hind limb surgery, the iliopsoas muscle is commonly tight or sore from compensation after lameness. This stretch will help relieve hip flexor muscle tension, which will in turn improve limb lowering and weight-bearing. The height of forelimb elevation should start low and then increase to the level that is comfortable and maintain hind paws to the ground. If the elevation is too high for the patient, they may be painful or lift the surgical leg and not benefit from this stretch. The object used for forelimb elevation can include a balance pad, exercise platform, low stair step, or other sturdy objects. Good traction is important to avoid slipping, and a yoga mat can be used over the surface.

WEEKS 2 TO 4

At this phase in recovery, goals are to improve weight-bearing, proprioception, and gaiting. Exercises in this phase include cavaletti rails, paw lifts, and figure eights. Range of motion transitions from PROM to more active range of motion . We can begin to increase slow-controlled leash walks to 10 to 15 minutes, with a harness or sling if needed. Stretches should be continued and can be advanced to side bend stretching to the hip level for patients agile enough. Height can be increased for step-up stretches to allow more hip extension.

Cavaletti exercises have many benefits and can easily be done using makeshift materials. A curtain tension rod can be placed in a hallway at desired height. Alternative objects that could be used include, broomstick handles, plastic pipes, or garden hose. The objects should be placed a distance of one stride length of the patient apart. The height should ideally start slightly above the dog's carpus.[10] The patient should be directed to walk slowly over the objects placing one paw at a time without hopping (**Fig. 4**). This will help with limb proprioception, improving stride length, joint range of motion, limb weight distribution, and balance. Low cavaletti exercise studied in kinematic motion analysis and found significant increase of flexion in elbow, carpal, stifle and tarsal joints, and extension in carpal and stifle joints.[11] This makes it an ideal exercise following stifle surgeries to improve the range of motion. Start this exercise with 10-15 repetitiions once daily.

Single leg paw lift exercise involves gently lifting one limb off the ground to shift more weight onto the desired limb. To shift more weight to the left hind limb, alternate between lifting the right hind limb and then the right forelimb (**Fig. 5**). The opposite can

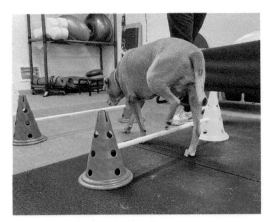

Fig. 4. Cavaletti rail exercise using cones and poles.

be done if the surgical limb is the right hind limb. Lifting a forelimb will shift weight to the diagonal hind limb. The limb should be gently lifted only 1 to 2 inches off the ground without over abduction or adduction. Each limb can be lifted for 5 to 15 seconds and 3 to 10 repetitions, 1 to 2 times daily.

Figure eight exercises can be added, which is easy to have clients perform at home by guiding the dog in a figure eight pattern around 2 marker objects. This exercise helps improve spine lateral flexion, proprioception, use of hind limb abductors and adductors and stability in directional transitions. Starting with cones farther apart for wide-based turns is ideal for smooth transitions and moving them closer as the dog progresses for 3 to 8 repetitions (**Fig. 6**).

WEEKS 4 TO 6

Goals are to improve strength, stability, and endurance. Exercise challenge is added in this phase with balance disc work, low incline walking, and sit to stands. Leash walk time can generally be increased to 15 to 20 minutes. The patient's ability and preinjury routine walking endurance should be considered.

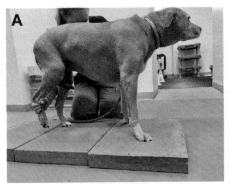
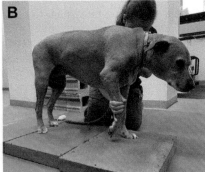

Fig. 5. Paw lift exercise (*A*)lifting right hind limb shifting to the left hind limb (*B*) Lifting right forelimb shifting weight to left hind limb (The opposite can be done if the right hind limb is the focus).

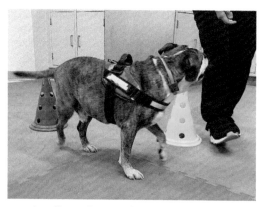

Fig. 6. Figure eight exercise allows alternate limb weight-bearing, lateral spine flexion, co-ordination, and balance work.

Weight shifting exercise can be advanced to stepping front limbs on a balance disc and holding a stand for 10 to 60 second sets (**Fig. 7**). The mild elevation of the front limbs will shift weight to the hind limbs and the balance challenge to the front limbs will elicit muscle contractions for stabilization in the hind limbs. This exercise may start by introducing the patient to the disc and reward them for placing a paw on the disc, gradually working up to both front paws on and holding the stand position. For some patients, a 10 to 20-second hold of this posture will be challenging enough to start, and for others, 60 seconds may easily be obtained; 1 to 4 repetitions.

Gentle low-incline walking can be included in outdoor excursions where available. Incline walking will increase hind limb weight-bearing and strength. Walking up the incline surface shifts the patient's center of gravity back increasing hind limb weight load. Walking up hill can be assumed to be helpful in strengthening the muscles involved in forward propulsion: biceps femoris, semitendinosus, and semimembranosus.[11]

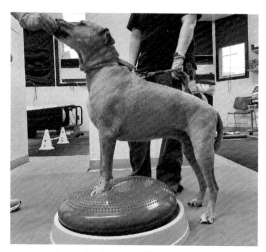

Fig. 7. Balance disc stand with forelimbs on shifting weight to hind limbs. The hind limbs should be centered squarely under the pelvis and forelimbs under the shoulders, whereas the head is directed slightly up.

Alternatively, side walking along a hill side with the surgical limb on the up side of the hill will engage more weight-bearing to this limb. Hill or side incline walking should be started slowly with a few minutes per walk session. If this is difficult or causes increase discomfort, it should be discontinued for the time being.

Sitting posture has often changed due to the reduced range of motion in the stifle, limb off loading, and compensatory muscular tension or discomfort. Patients may side sit onto one hip, rolling their pelvis under and extending hind limbs forward. This posture will place strain on the low back and reduce hind limb engagement when rising, relying more on front limbs to pull up to stand. Start with sitting posture work when safe and comfortable. For most patients that falls in week 4 of recovery. Dogs with advanced joint disease may be uncomfortable and limited in stifle flexion. Sitting to the ground may not be possible or comfortable. If they are able to partially lower to a sit a towel roll or bolster may be placed under the pelvis to allow the dog to sit with decreased stifle flexion in a more normal square sitting position. The elevated sitting posture is also good for dogs not fully able to sit to the ground for sit to stand exercises. In a square sit position, the tarsi are under the hips and the lumbar spine is extended. Generally, manual assistance is needed to achieve this because it is not a natural feeling for a dog to sit on objects. For dogs that are able to sit fully to the ground but are placing the surgical limb lateral, a wall can be used as a guide. By having the patient sit with the affected limb against a wall or between 2 objects, a square sitting posture is reinforced. Reinforcement of this posture can simply be started by just having the pet sit in this position for a few minutes at a time.

Starting from a sitting position in good form, sit to stand exercises can done for 3 to 10 repetitions (**Fig. 8**). This allows the sit to stand to be an effective exercise because the pets are placed in a position where they can engage their hind limbs to push up to stand. This is particularly helpful for weakened quadriceps muscles and also engages biceps femoris, semitendinosus, semimembranosus, gastrocnemius, and gluteal muscles. Sit to stand exercises can start after the subacute phase; however, waiting until 4 weeks postoperative for patients recovering from a TPLO or patella luxation correction is advised because this exercise could potentially cause patella tendon strain if started too soon.

Once the patient is able to sit and stand readily and with ease, the challenge can be increased by placing the forelimbs on low elevation to put more workload on the hind limbs. Initially start with forelimbs on a low firm cushion and advance to forelimbs on a balance disc or low platform such as an aerobics stepper. A bolster can again be used under the pelvis for those dogs that have limited stifle flexion. Repetitions can increase to 5 to 15 depending on the patient's ability.

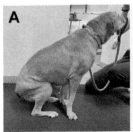 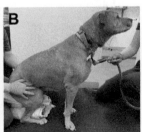 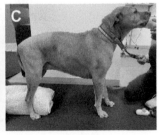

Fig. 8. (*A*) The dog is unable to fully sit due to reduced stifle flexion. (*B*) Improved sitting position with a bolster under the pelvis. From this position, the hocks can be seated under the hips. (*C*) The dog can then rise to a stand with effective hind limb push off.

WEEKS 6 TO 8

During this time in recovery, patients are usually rechecking with the surgeon and radiographs are repeated as recommended. More dynamic exercises can usually be started past this point if the healing progress is going well. Goals are to continue to regain muscle mass in the surgical limb, core strength for stability and prevention of injury. Exercises that may be added in this phase include side and backwards stepping, diagonal paw lifts, all limbs on balance surfaces and stair steps. Leash walks can continue to increase by an additional 5 minutes per week to reach their goal walk time.

This is a good time to reevaluate any areas that are lagging in recovery such as muscle mass, range of motion, weight-bearing distribution, or compensatory issues in areas that took additional workload during recovery. Addressing this now is advisable before moving on to full recovery and return to normal activity to avoid further injury. Areas identified that need further work can guide the exercise program during these weeks of recovery. Continue restriction of off leash play and running but the intensity and duration of exercises and walks can be increased for those cases progressing as expected.

Backwards and side stepping can be instituted to engage different muscle groups. Backwards stepping will engage semitendinosus, semimembranosus, and gluteal muscles.[12] These can be done by standing on the side of the pet for side stepping (**Fig. 9**) or in front guiding them back for backwards, taking several steps in each direction. Start with 10 steps in each direction for 1 to 5 repetitions. For those patients that are able, side stepping can be advanced to placing forelimbs on a balance disc and pivoting to side step their hind limbs around the disc. The additional balance challenge will increase weight-bearing and stability in the hind limbs.

Core strength exercises can be added to the routine to help with injury prevention as the patient prepares for return to activity. Paw lift exercises can be advanced to diagonal forelimb and hind limb lifts (2-leg stands) for those dogs who are ready to advance from the single leg paw lift to 2-leg paw lifts (3-leg stands). Forelimbs on a balance disc and hind limbs on a cushion, or another balance disc, can also be used as a core strength exercise (**Fig. 10**).

Stair exercise can be a beneficial exercise in hind limb strengthening, range of motion and proprioception. Quadriceps and gluteal muscles are strengthened during push off.[13] Kinematic analysis comparing stair ascent to level land trotting found all hind limb joints had a greater joint motion on stairs. Greater extension of the hip

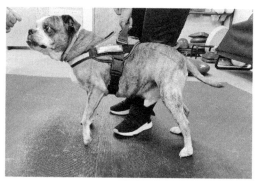

Fig. 9. Side stepping exercise to engage adductor and abductor muscles. Start by facing a lateral side of the dog and walking toward them to guide side stepping.

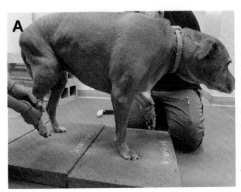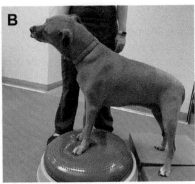

Fig. 10. Core strength. (*A*) alternate paw lifts (*B*) advanced balance stands with all 4 limbs on balance equipment.

and stifle and maximum flexion of the stifle and tarsal joints were also noted in stair ascent.[14] Stair reintroduction should be included in those cases where taking stairs was a preinjury activity and when appropriate for the animal. Considering any other concurrent orthopedic or neurologic concerns where this exercise should not be advised. Stairs that have good traction, such as carpet, rubber mats or outdoor concrete should be used to avoid slipping during the recovery phase. The pet should be guided on leash to take one stair at a time without leaping and bounding. If the dog is comfortable with this, start with 1 to 3 repetitions of a short stair set (8–12 steps) during their exercises.

BEYOND 8 WEEKS

The final phase of recovery is usually after 8 weeks when a slow return to normal activity is granted. This decision should involve the surgeon to ensure that healing is adequate to resume these activities. Osteotomies may not be fully healed until 8 to 12 weeks and for these patients, caution should be continued avoiding high-level activities. Healing must be fully complete and strength gained before resuming sporting activities. The slow return should take 4 to 8 weeks or longer for those animals who previously had a higher level of activity. Exercises during this phase will be directed based on the patient's preinjury normal activity and goals.

Warming up before activity can help reduce injury. This can include a 5-minute walk, some stretches, or cavaletti exercises. Trotting and running should only be started in slow controlled increments before short sets of off leash activity are allowed. It is advisable to choose a small confined area without other dogs initially. If increasing the activity causes discomfort or soreness, it should be reduced to the tolerated level and worked back up more slowly.

ADDITIONAL CONSIDERATIONS

Periodic assessments should be done to ensure healing and progression is at an appropriate level before advancing to the next stage of exercise. A review of available evidence for rehabilitation following CCL repair surgery recommended that rehabilitation programs should be based on patient progress, individual assessment, and on fundamental principles of tissue healing.[15] Concurrent conditions that may cause pain or limit the patient's ability should always be considered. Pain control should be assessed throughout recovery using medications and pain-relieving modalities as needed. Modalities commonly used in rehabilitation therapy may be incorporated when available to provide adjunctive pain control such as laser, pulsed electromagnetic therapy, electrical stimulation, and acupuncture. Weight management should be included as part of the recovery process, particularly if the patient is over ideal weight. Obesity will place additional stress on the joints and decrease the patient's ability to exercise. Advising on supportive devices and home modifications should be included when needed. This may include slings, harnesses, ramps, traction runners, or gripping paw covers to help avoid slipping injury.

SUMMARY

Therapy exercises can provide improved functional outcome for dogs following CCL repair surgery. Benefits include improved range of motion, proprioception, muscle mass, strength, balance, endurance, and prevention of injury. Even basic exercises can provide benefits, and these can often be done in the home setting with instruction given to clients. Exercises should be based appropriately for the phase of recovery, the ability of the patient, and any concurrent medical problems.

CLINICS CARE POINTS

- Communication with the surgeon is important to be aware of any special patient concerns and progress.
- Dog and pet owner's ability and mobility should be considered when choosing appropriate home exercises.
- Frequency and repetitions should be tailored for the individual patient; start with one set of a low number of repetitions and gradually work up.
- Keeping the time commitment short will increase compliance for home exercises, such as 15 to 20 minutes per session.

SUPPLEMENTARY DATA

Supplementary data related to this article can be found online at https://doi.org/10.1016/j.cvsm.2023.02.013.

DECLARATION OF INTERESTS

No interests to declare.

REFERENCES

1. Spinella G, Arcamone G, Valentini S. Cranial cruciate ligament rupture in dogs: review on biomechanics, etiopathogenic factors and rehabilitation. Vet Sci 2021;8:1–22.
2. Alvarez LX, Repac JA, Kirkby-Shaw K, et al. Systematic review of postoperative rehabilitation interventions after cranial cruciate ligament surgery in dogs. Vet Surg 2022;51:233–43.
3. Marsolais GS, Dvorak G, Conzemius M. Effects of postoperative rehabilitation on limb function after cranial cruciate ligament repair in dogs. J Am Vet Med Assoc 2002;220:1325–30.

4. Monk M, Preston CA, McGowan CM. Effects of early intensive postoperative physiotherapy on limb function after tibial plateau leveling osteotomy in dogs with deficiency of the cranial cruciate ligament. Am J Vet Res 2006;67:529–36.

5. Millis DL, Drum M, Levine D. Therapeutic exercises: early limb use exercises. In: Millis DL, Levine D, editors. Canine rehabilitation and physical therapy. 2nd edition. St. Louis, MO: Elsevier; 2014. p. 495–505.

6. Eiermann J, Kirkby-Shaw K, Evans RB, et al. Recommendations for rehabilitation after surgical treatment of cranial cruciate ligament disease in dogs: A 2017 survey of veterinary practitioners. Vet Surg 2020;49:80–7.

7. Baltzer WI. Rehabilitation of companion animals following orthopedic surgery. N Z Vet J 2020;68:157–67.

8. Nadler SF, Weingand K, Kruse RJ. The physiologic basis and clinical applications of cryotherapy and thermotherapy for the pain practitioner. Pain Physician 2004; 7:395–9.

9. Davidson JR, Kerwin S. Common orthopedic conditions and their physical rehabilitation. In: Millis DL, Levine D, editors. Canine rehabilitation and physical therapy. 2nd edition. St. Louis, MO: Elsevier; 2014. p. 543–81.

10. Drum MG, Marcellin-Little DJ, Davis MS. Principles and applications of therapeutic exercises for small animals. Vet Clin North Am Small Anim Pract 2015;45: 73–90.

11. Holler PJ, Brazda V, Lewy E, et al. Kinematic motion analysis of the joints of the forelimbs and hind limbs of dogs during walking exercise regimens. Am J Vet Res 2010;71:734–40.

12. Medina C. Guidelines to home exercises and lifestyle modifications for common small animal orthopedic conditions. Vet Clin North Am Small Anim Pract 2022;52: 1021–32.

13. Millis DL, Drum M, Levine D. Therapeutic exercises: joint motion, strengthening, endurance, and speed exercises. In: Millis DL, Levine D, editors. Canine rehabilitation and physical therapy. 2nd edition. St. Louis, MO: Elsevier; 2014. p. 506–25.

14. Durant AM, Millis DL, Headrick JF. Kinematics of stair ascent in healthy dogs. Vet Comp Orthop Traumatol 2011;24:99–105.

15. Kirkby-Shaw K, Alvarez L, Foster SA, et al. Fundamental principles of rehabilitation and musculoskeletal tissue healing. Vet Surg 2020;49:22–32.

Rehabilitation to Return-to-Work for Working Dogs

Meghan T. Ramos, VMD[a],*, Brian D. Farr, DVM, MSTR, DACVPM[b],
Cynthia M. Otto, DVM, PhD, DACVECC, DACVSMR[a]

KEYWORDS

- Rehabilitation • Return-to-work • Musculoskeletal • Sports medicine
- Working dogs

KEY POINTS

- Working dogs are at risk of deconditioning with activity restriction of greater than 2 weeks.
- Communication and management of objective benchmarks with the handler are critical for the determination of clearance to return-to-work, retirement, or career alterations.
- Return-to-work for a working dog is considered a success if the dog can perform all career-related activity safely and proficiently.

INTRODUCTION

Definition of a Working Dog

Recently, the American Animal Hospital Association published guidelines for the veterinary care of working, assistance, and therapy animals.[1] Although all three types of dogs have unique care requirements, this article will focus on working dogs, which specifically include scent detection and protection dogs. The physical requirements of these canine athletes vary with the physical work that they perform and the environment in which that work is performed. The veterinary team providing rehabilitation for these dogs needs to be aware of the specific job requirements so that they can focus their plan to maximize the dog's potential to return-to-work and minimize future injuries.

Detection dogs are employed to use their noses to find trained odors/scents, but what they are trained to detect and the physical environment in which they work can be highly variable. See **Table 1** for common scent detection careers. The physical requirements of a detection dog will be determined by whether they are searching indoors or outdoors, on leash or off leash, and in controlled environments or exposed

[a] Penn Vet Working Dog Center, Clinical Sciences and Advanced Medicine, School of Veterinary Medicine, University of Pennsylvania, 3401 Grays Ferry Avenue, Philadelphia, PA 19146, USA;
[b] Department of Defense Military Working Dog Veterinary Service, Joint Base San Antonio – Lackland Air Force Base, San Antonio, TX, USA
* Corresponding author.
E-mail address: megramos@upenn.edu

Vet Clin Small Anim 53 (2023) 869–878
https://doi.org/10.1016/j.cvsm.2023.02.014
0195-5616/23/© 2023 Elsevier Inc. All rights reserved.

Table 1
Summary of working dog career types, ownership, and environmental considerations

Dog	Agency	Trained Odor	Environment
Bomb dog or explosive detection canine (EDC)	Law enforcement, Alcohol, Tobacco, Firearms and Explosives (ATF), Department of Defense, Transportation Security Administration	Explosives including home-made explosives	Indoors (e.g., airports, shipping, buildings) Outdoor (eg, vehicle search, perimeter search, route clearance)
Drug dog or narcotics detection dog	Law enforcement, private companies, Department of Homeland Security, Customs and Border Protection	Various illicit drugs (not limited to narcotics)	Indoors (eg, packages, buildings) Outdoors (eg, vehicle search, hidden caches)
Arson dog or Accelerant (ignitable liquid) detection dog	Fire departments, ATF, insurance companies	Ignitable liquids (fire starters)	Fire scenes (after fires extinguished)
Agriculture or Beagle Brigade	United States Department of Agriculture	Illegally imported produce, meats, cheeses	Airports (international arrivals), Ports
Bed bug dog/pest detection dog	Commercial companies, private individuals	Cyanix (bed bugs)	Indoors: Houses, hotels, schools, airplanes
Conservation dog	Nonprofits, companies, Customs and Border Protection	Invasive, endangered species, smuggled wildlife/products	Indoors—screening shipments, baggage Outdoors—environment dependent on species detected
Urban/disaster search and rescue dog	Fire departments, police departments, Federal Emergency Management Agency, private citizens (volunteers), law enforcement, National Guard	Live find: concealed humans Human remains detection (aka cadaver dog)	Disaster settings—collapsed buildings, infrastructure
Wilderness/area search and rescue dog	Private citizens, law enforcement	Live find: lost humans Human remains detection	Wilderness, urban, suburban, water
Pipeline leak detection dogs	companies	Natural Gas	Outdoors

to variations in temperature, humidity, and wind. Furthermore, work: rest cycles will impact the need for physical stamina. Most detection dogs will work for 30 to 60 minutes followed by a similar period of rest. Dogs which are required to traverse uneven surfaces (eg, search and rescue dogs [both urban and wilderness], conservation dogs, and some bomb and drug dogs) will require a higher degree of physical fitness, strength, stamina, balance, and proprioception than dogs working in more controlled environments such as airports or cargo shipping centers. Most detection dogs are required to search at different heights; for example, while searching a vehicle, they may need to stand on their hind legs to reach areas, or while searching inside buildings they may be required to search under desks and high on shelves. This physical requirement, particularly for searching high, results in the quadruped dog becoming more like a biped; bearing all its weight on its hind limbs and subjecting its lumbosacral spine to increased vertical forces as well as repetitive flexion and extension. Detection dogs which search for human scent (live or deceased) often work in challenging environments. Disaster search dogs respond to natural and humanmade disasters and typically must navigate collapsed buildings and urban debris in all types of weather conditions. Typically, wide area or wilderness search dogs and some conservation dogs work in more rural or wilderness areas where they encounter difficult terrain, natural (eg, water, rocks, wildlife) and humanmade hazards (eg, barbed wire, fences).

Protection dogs include military working dogs, law enforcement patrol dogs, private protection dogs, and livestock guarding dogs. Most law enforcement patrol dogs are considered dual purpose in that they are trained to perform a detection task (usually explosives or narcotics) and patrol work. Criminal apprehension is a major part of the law enforcement canine's job. The dog is trained to track humans, find discarded evidence (containing human scent), and apprehend and restrain suspects. Although, historically, these dogs have been referred to as "attack dogs", it is more accurate to describe their work as controlled aggression. The dogs will chase and bite a fleeing suspect, but the goal of the bite is to stop and restrain the individual, not to engage in an attack or repeated biting. These dogs require power, stamina, and strength. Most agencies do not focus on proprioception or balance in their training but incorporating it into a rehabilitation or fitness plan may help prevent future injuries. Law enforcement canines are typically owned by the law enforcement agency, whether it is federal, state, or local.

Some organizations will house working dogs in kennels, but it is common for many programs to have dogs live with their handlers. The housing environment is an important consideration in rehabilitation plans. Kennel housing may lead to unique repetitive motion injuries and may make home rehabilitation more challenging due to limited access to the dog.

Why Return-To-Work is Important

The purpose of rehabilitation for companion dogs is "return-to-function" or regaining the ability to perform as many of the common daily tasks as possible. These tasks include rising from a sit, ascending and descending stairs, posturing to eliminate, and walking without discomfort. For many companion dogs, the goal is also to regain the ability to perform as many elective activities as possible like playing with another animal, swimming, or playing with a person.

Working dogs undergoing rehabilitation require an additional return-to-work period as their jobs demand slightly more (eg, agriculture detection) to far more (eg, dual-purpose law enforcement) physical ability than is expected of companion dogs. There are numerous reasons that working dogs benefit from a return-to-work program, however, before designing a program, the rehabilitation professional must have a clear understanding of the dog's job requirements and physical risks. Just like any other professional athlete, working dogs' jobs require a level of fitness to safely and effectively perform their duties. Incremental and targeted strength training combined with objective measures of canine fitness as related to their specific work requirements can help reduce the risk of injury. Although return-to-work is the goal, an objective assessment will also allow clear communication if a dog is no longer capable of performing its job safely and effectively. In addition, advocating for a return-to-work period will help demonstrate the veterinary team's knowledge of the dog's job, communicate respect for the demands of the job, and develop rapport with the handler and owning/supporting agency. **Box 1** provides several key reasons for including a return-to-work period in the rehabilitation of a working dog.

It is well-recognized that conditioning requires months whereas deconditioning happens in weeks. Working dogs are professional athletes and any prolonged interruption in their activity can lead to deconditioning (and often weight gain). Even if the dog does not have an injury traditionally warranting rehabilitation, a return-to-work plan should be included for any working dog who has experienced a gap in training or work. See **Table 2** for common medical and handler reasons to initiate a return-to-work plan. One of the first components of the return-to-work assessment should include body condition score and then functional fitness.

Identifying Expectations

In addition to understanding the requirements of the dog, working dog clients have unique communication requirements. For working dogs which are owned by departments or agencies, financial decisions and communication about prognosis and recovery timelines will need to include the relevant supervisors in addition to the handler. The working dog handler should be actively involved in all assessments and treatments. Working dogs, although highly trained, are often easily aroused which can make them challenging to handle. Incorporating the handler in the examination will reduce the stress for the dog, handler, and veterinary team and thereby facilitate cooperative care. The handler will often be able to provide the appropriate commands so the dog can perform exercises or be examined. The rehabilitation clinician should be prepared to premedicate some working dogs (eg, gabapentin and trazadone) to facilitate the examination and therapeutic interventions. Many working dogs, especially protection dogs, may require a muzzle during examination or rehabilitation visits; the veterinary team should not hesitate to request a dog be muzzled. Even with a muzzle, the use of positive reinforcement and food rewards can be implemented. As with any client, it is important to discuss the use of food with the handler to ensure that there are no allergies or contraindications for use of food. Some handlers may be

---

Box 1
Key reasons for including a return-to-work period in the rehabilitation of a working dog

Regaining lost fitness to ensure task performance

Confirming regained fitness through assessment

Reducing the risk of reinjury or injury to another area

Guiding appropriate inclusion of task training (eg, detection at nose level vs while standing on the hind legs) as physical ability increases

Determining suitability for work vs guiding career change or retirement decisions

Rebuilding handler and owning/supporting agency confidence in the dog's abilities

Table 2 Common medical and handler reasons to initiate a return-to-work plan	
Reasons to initiate a return-to-work plan	
Medical reasons	Muscular injuries e.g., muscle strains or tears Tendon or ligament injuries e.g., ligament sprains, tendinopathy Orthopedic injuries e.g., bone fractures, joint injuries/disease Wounds e.g., lacerations, Recovery from elective procedures like prophylactic gastropexy Recovery from emergency procedures like laparotomy for foreign body removal Extended illness or hospitalization

Non-medical reasons	Handler injury or illness
	Handler non-availability due to attending non-dog training or
	    a personal situation
	Seasonal work like avalanche rescue dogs without off-season
	    sustainment

reluctant to use food, but they can often be educated as to the benefits of this low-stress approach to benefit their dog's recovery. Some handlers may suggest that a toy reward is preferred, but often the toy is too stimulating for the dog to remain relaxed and compliant.

One of the first steps in establishing a rehabilitation plan is to determine the therapeutic goals. For a working dog, these goals will be dependent on the type of job and the expectations of the agency/handler. Clear communication is essential. Some handlers may have limited ability to perform at-home exercises. Some agencies may have unrealistic expectations for the dog to return-to-work quickly. The rehabilitation professional needs to educate the canine team about the healing process, tissue strength, and the risk of repeated injury if the plan is rushed. One of the greatest challenges in rehabilitation for working dogs is the discussion of whether the dog can safely and successfully return-to-work. Working dogs are highly motivated and retirement may not easily suit their personality or the handler's lifestyle. Sometimes, it is possible for a dog to continue working, but at a less intensive job. For example, a dual-purpose dog may be able to continue detection work but no longer participate in protection work.

Establishment of Timelines

The rehabilitative approach to a working dog recovery plan consists of four distinct sequential phases: activity restriction, rehabilitation, return-to-work, and maintenance.[2] The timeline for progression through each phase is dependent on location and degree of injury, treatment intervention, prior health status of the dog, and compliance of the handler to follow activity modifications and restrictions.[3,4] Similar to a professional human athlete, any disruption of an athletic routine requires a comprehensive plan beyond daily tasks or low-intensity exercise.[5,6]

Return-to-work for a working dog is considered a success if the dog can perform all career-related activities safely and proficiently.[2] Depending on the career of the dog, this could include navigating dangerous terrain, pursuing a criminal, or demonstrating that an event venue is free of explosives as highlighted in **Table 1**. The location and extent of the injury are important in determining a realistic timeline for the dog to return-to-work. At a minimum, the injury timeline will follow the general principles of healing and strength of the tissue type (ie, muscle, tendon, bone, ligament). For example, a muscle tear may take 6 months for the tissue to heal.[3] This healing does not account for re-establishing stability and strength within the muscle that will be required for a working dog to return-to-work. Depending on the location of the muscle tear, it may not be vital to the dog's daily work tasks or all the work tasks and therefore the dog may be able to return to certain work-related activities such as obedience or controlled on-leash odor detection before the 6-month timeline. As illustrated throughout this article, a plethora of information must be considered before clearing a dog for active duty.

When the Transition from Rehabilitation to Return-To-Work Occurs

The goals of rehabilitation in companion dogs are pain mitigation, re-establishment of basic mobility (ie, sitting, standing, laying down, walking), and increased quality of life.[3,4,7,8] The transition from rehabilitation to return-to-work occurs after the working dog has met the goals of traditional rehabilitation.[2,8] Advanced exercises cannot safely be pursued without the foundation of good posture in sit, down, or stance positions. Similarly, many working dog careers require the dog to have enough strength and stability to hold its body weight as a tripod or bipod. Return-to-work protocols are focused on re-establishing or enhancing proprioception, strength, stability, muscular endurance, and cardiorespiratory endurance through advanced therapeutic exercise and career-specific tasks. An example of an advanced traditional rehabilitation exercise is the canine squat which is a more challenging sit-to-stand (**Fig. 1**). Dynamic plyometric exercises (eg, jumping onto a platform from a sit or down position), core strengthening exercises (eg, plank), and dynamic movement targeting the critical muscles used in career-specific tasks (eg, pivot, backing up, tugging with a toy, and sprinting) are utilized in return-to-work programs to mimic career-related tasks (**Fig. 2**). Before progressing or continuing any exercise, veterinarians and rehabilitation specialists should monitor the posture of the dog during the exercises.

The Process of Creating a Program

Defining the extent of injury, documenting any unique financial constraints, and knowledge of the physical requirements of the dog's career are the first steps in the creation of a return to program for a working dog. The outlined decision tree in **Fig. 3** provides a practical guide to a baseline return-to-work program. Clear communication of the timeline and benchmarks of success are important for objective assessment of the dog to return-to-work.

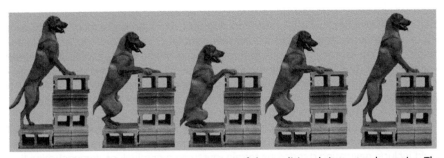

Fig. 1. The canine squat exercise is a progression of the traditional sit-to-stand exercise. The squat builds on the hindlimb strength and stability of the sit-to-stand by increasing the distribution of body weight to the hindlimbs by elevating the forelimbs. The dog is asked to sit while maintaining the forelimbs on the platform into a square sit, followed by an explosive propulsion to stand.

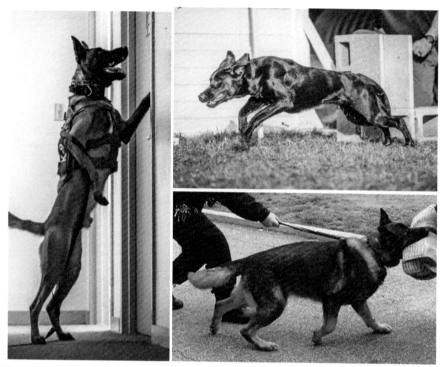

Fig. 2. Examples of dynamic movement targeting the critical muscles used in career-specific tasks. The left photo demonstrates a "paws-up" activity in which a dog moves into a biped position, placing majority of its weight onto the hindlimbs. The top right photo highlights a still frame of a working dog sprinting. The bottom right photo demonstrates a tug exercise with all four limbs remaining in contact with the ground. All photos highlight movements that are performed in a working dog's career.

The Benchmarks of Success

Benchmarks are objective measures of a return-to-work program related to the dog's career. The objective measurements are used to assess and deduce the dog's capabilities to safely return-to-work. Examples of objective measurements are highlighted in **Table 3**. The benchmarks are helpful in communication and monitoring of progress for the handlers, trainers, departments, and internal veterinary care team. If a dog fails to meet all or some of the objective benchmarks, the decision to retire or alter the dog's career is more straightforward. Objectivity may help relieve any guilt or emotions related to retirement or a scaled-back career for both the handler and veterinarian.

The Lifelong Program

A working dog completing the return-to-work portion of a rehabilitation program should then begin a lifelong fitness program. Canine rehabilitation practitioners should encourage this continuation for several reasons. First, if the original reason for seeking care was a potentially preventable neuromusculoskeletal issue (eg, muscular strain), ongoing fitness training should lower the risk of recurrence. In these cases, handlers who were not performing preventive practices (eg, warm-up routines) are likely now receptive to including them. For issues with residual and lifelong deficiencies (eg, stifle

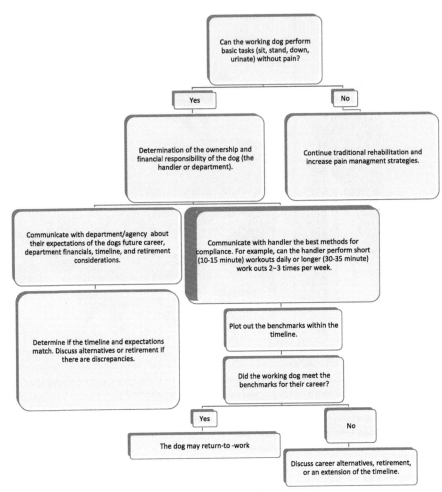

Fig. 3. A practical guide to a baseline return-to-work program.

degenerative joint disease following cranial cruciate ligament disease and tibial plateau leveling osteotomy), continued fitness training can minimize inevitable imbalance and provide early notice of compensation. Furthermore, handlers completing the return-to-work phase are typically much more aware of their dog's movement, especially in areas directly related to the original issue. Continuing this awareness through ongoing fitness training may provide earlier awareness of recurrence or of new problems. Finally, handlers who put the work in through the entire return-to-function and return-to-work phases can now leverage that experience and enhanced relationship with their dog into an ongoing fitness program. Handlers like this may even become the model for performance, fitness, and preventive care and create positive change within their agency or organization.

This ongoing fitness training should also bring the rehabilitation practitioner into the cohort supporting the working dog team. There, alongside the trainer and agency/organization leadership, the rehabilitation practitioner can advocate for the dog's health, welfare, and performance. Leveraging the trust gained and rapport built through the rehabilitation process, the practitioner can check in with the dog and handler at

Table 3
Objective benchmarks of a return-to-work program related to the dog's career

Objective Benchmark	Recommended Objective Benchmarks to Return-to-Work Based on Career		
	Law Enforcement Dual purpose	Search and Rescue-Urban	Single Purpose Odor Detection
Perform the squat with appropriate posture at shoulder height without pain for seven repetitions twice a week	Highly Recommended	Highly recommended	Recommended
Sprint (25 m) for five repetitions without lameness or pain	Highly recommended	Highly recommended	Recommended
Tug with forelimbs elevated for 2 minutes without compromised posture	Highly recommended	Recommended	Recommended
Tug with all limbs on the ground elevated for 2 minutes without compromised posture	Highly recommended	Highly recommended	Consider
Jump over minimum 2-foot height without pain or instability	Highly recommended	Highly recommended	Recommended
Perform Plank for 1 minute	Highly recommended	Highly recommended	Highly recommended
Maintain Paws-up position (full hip extension) for 30 seconds with even weight distribution on both hindlimbs	Highly recommended	Highly recommended	Highly recommended

The objective measurements are used to assess and deduce the dog's capabilities to safely return-to-work.

scheduled sessions and accurately convey the current status and expected future performance to the dog team's leadership.

DISCLOSURE

The authors do not have any commercial or financial conflicts of interest regarding the material presented in this article. The authors (Ramos and Otto) are employed with the Penn Vet Working Dog Center (PVWDC). The PVWDC currently receives funding from Pennsylvania Emergency Management Agency, Pennsylvania Game Commission, National Institutes of Health, Department of Homeland Security, United States Department of Agriculture, Kleberg Foundation, and Zoetis. The sports medicine and rehabilitation residency at the PVWDC at the time of publication is sponsored by Dechra. Donors to the PVWDC are Dechra, Nestle-Purina, Royal Canin, Nutramax, Boehringer-Ingelheim, Merial, Merck, and Respond Systems. The PVWDC was previously funded by Nestle-Purina, Virox, Red Arch Cultural Heritage Law & Policy Research Foundation. The views expressed are those of the author (Farr) and do not reflect the official policy or position of the US Army, Department of Defense, or the US Government.

CLINICS CARE POINTS

- Working dog rehabilitation consists of four distinct sequential phases: activity restriction, general rehabilitation, return-to-work, and maintenance fitness and conditioning.
- Deconditioning happens within 2 weeks of inactivity, and working dogs which are on extended activity restriction for any reason should undergo rehabilitation and return-to-work exercise programs.
- Objective benchmarks within a return-to-work program are critical for the determination of clearance to work, retirement, or career alterations for the working dog.

REFERENCES

1. Otto CM, Darling T, Murphy L, et al. AAHA Working, Assistance, and Therapy Dog Guidelines. J Am Anim Hosp Assoc 2021;57(6):253–77.
2. Ramos MT, Farr BD, Otto CM. Sports Medicine and Rehabilitation in Working Dogs. Vet Clin North Am Small Anim Pract 2021;51(4):859–76.
3. Kirkby Shaw K, Alvarez L, Foster SA, et al. Fundamental principles of rehabilitation and musculoskeletal tissue healing. Vet Surg 2020;49(1):22–32.
4. Dycus DL, Levine D, Marcellin-Little DJ. Physical Rehabilitation for the Management of Canine Hip Dysplasia. Vet Clin North Am Small Anim Pract 2017;47(4):823–50.
5. Dijkstra HP, Pollock N, Chakraverty R, et al. Managing the health of the elite athlete: a new integrated performance health management and coaching model. Br J Sports Med 2014;48(7):523–31.
6. Faigenbaum AD, Myer GD. Resistance training among young athletes: safety, efficacy and injury prevention effects. Br J Sports Med 2010;44(1):56–63.
7. Frye C, Carr BJ, Lenfest M, et al. Canine Geriatric Rehabilitation: Considerations and Strategies for Assessment, Functional Scoring, and Follow Up. Front Vet Sci 2022;9:842458.
8. Zink MC, Van Dyke JB. Canine sports medicine and rehabilitation. John Wiley & Sons, Incorporated; 2013. Available at: http://ebookcentral.proquest.com/lib/upenn-ebooks/detail.action?docID=1132530. Accessed September 17, 2020.

Feline Osteoarthritis Management

Kelly Deabold, DVM, CCRV CVA[a], Christina Montalbano, VMD, DACVSMR, CCRP, CVA[b],
Erin Miscioscia, DVM, DACVSMR, CVA[a],*

KEYWORDS

- Feline • Osteoarthritis • Integrative veterinary medicine • Rehabilitation
- Acupuncture • Nutrition • Supplement

KEY POINTS

- Feline osteoarthritis (OA) is common, with prevalence increasing with age. The most commonly affected joints include the elbow, hip, stifle, and shoulder; degenerative changes to the thoracolumbar spine are also common. Clinical signs are often vague and a combination of owner questionnaires, orthopedic examination, and radiography are recommended for identification.
- An integrative and multimodal approach to feline OA management is recommended to maintain quality of life. Considerations include anti-inflammatory and analgesic medications, dietary modifications, nutraceuticals, environmental modifications, and physical rehabilitation.
- Acupuncture and regenerative medicine may also be considered, although additional high-quality studies are indicated for these in feline OA.

BACKGROUND

Prevalence of Feline Osteoarthritis and Commonly Affected Joints

Osteoarthritis (OA) of the cat is a common disease, which may cause subtle changes in a cat's behavior but significantly affect quality of life (QOL). Reports of prevalence of OA in cat populations vary widely from 22% to 92%.[1–5] It is frequently considered a primary or idiopathic disease in cats[3,6] with a significant association between increasing age and the presence of radiographic signs of OA.[1–3,5,6] One study of cats aged older than 12 years found 90% of cats in this population had radiographic signs of OA.[4] Secondary OA is most commonly due to fractures or hip dysplasia.[6] Feline joints that are most commonly affected include elbows, hips, and to a lesser extent stifles and shoulders.[1–3,5,6] Bilateral joint disease is common.[1] Degenerative changes to the spine

[a] Department of Comparative, Diagnostic and Population Medicine, College of Veterinary Medicine, University of Florida, 2015 SW 16th Avenue, Gainesville, FL 32608, USA; [b] NorthStar VETS, 315 Robbinsville-Allentown Road, Robbinsville, NJ 08691, USA
* Corresponding author.
E-mail address: emiscioscia@ufl.edu

Vet Clin Small Anim 53 (2023) 879–896
https://doi.org/10.1016/j.cvsm.2023.02.015
vetsmall.theclinics.com

are also common, with reports of approximately 40% of cats having spondylosis deformans in the thoracic, lumbar, or lumbosacral spine.[1,7]

Diagnosis of Feline Osteoarthritis

Physical examination findings
Orthopedic and neurologic examination in cats is challenging in the veterinary environment and may be low yielding in the identification of OA. A quiet environment should be available, with a dedicated room for examination of cats when possible. The room should offer opportunities for cats to jump, and lack areas where cats could hide. Cats should be allowed to exit their carriers voluntarily, or should be gently removed to minimize discomfort and stress before examination. Examination may be performed with the cat remaining in its carrier with the top removed or through a top-opening door when feasible. Assessment of the cat's posture, gait, jumping ability, and other movements should be assessed before joint manipulations when possible. Nervous cats may adopt a crouched posture and refuse to ambulate, obscuring meaningful information. For this reason, owner-provided home videos are advantageous to allow observation of movement when walking on flat surfaces, on stairs, and jumping onto furniture in a stress-free environment. Regardless of whether gait analysis is performed in hospital or through home-video assessment, lameness is an uncommon finding.[1,2,6] Joint pain, crepitus, joint effusion, joint thickening, and abnormal range of motion (ROM) are hallmarks of OA in dogs but not all are consistent findings in feline OA.[8] Rather, palpation and goniometry may be more useful as a screening tool to identify joints that are likely unaffected by OA because lack of pain and higher ROM measurements tend to predict radiographically normal joints.[8] Whole limb manipulations can be assessed initially, with individual joint assessment performed where pain or abnormal ROM is identified. Assessment for spinal pain should follow joint evaluation; further neurologic assessment may be unreliable in a hospital setting even in neurologically normal cats.[9]

Radiographic findings
Where OA is suspected, survey orthogonal radiographs should be performed for confirmation and further characterization. Hallmark radiographic findings in cats differ from those in dogs, with joint effusion, osteophytes, and subchondral bone changes seen less frequently and periarticular new bone formation and joint-associated mineralization noted most commonly (**Figs. 1–3**).[10]

Subjective Assessment of Osteoarthritis Impairment

Clinical metrology instruments (CMIs) are questionnaires completed by the owner to evaluate changes in behavior and mobility in the home environment. These questionnaires are suggested as diagnostic tools for OA in cats, as well as to monitor response to treatment. The Feline Musculoskeletal Pain Index (FMPI) is the most developed tool to date assessing activity, pain intensity, and overall QOL. The FMPI is repeatable and reliable in identifying normal cats versus those affected by pain from OA, although it is unable to discriminate OA disease severity and has not been validated for monitoring response to treatment.[11,12] For this purpose, client-specific outcome measure (CSOM) questionnaires may better characterize impairment in individual cats and allow monitoring of treatment response.[13]

Objective Assessment of Osteoarthritis Impairment

Several methods of objective mobility impairment quantification in cats with OA have been assessed. These methods are typically reserved for research and are not likely

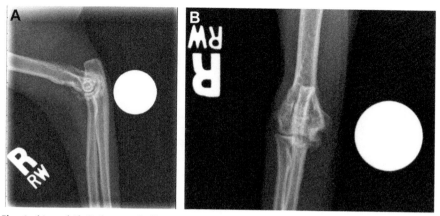

Fig. 1. (A and B) Orthogonal elbow radiographs of a 15-year-old female spayed Domestic Shorthair (DSH) demonstrating moderate right elbow periarticular osseous proliferation.

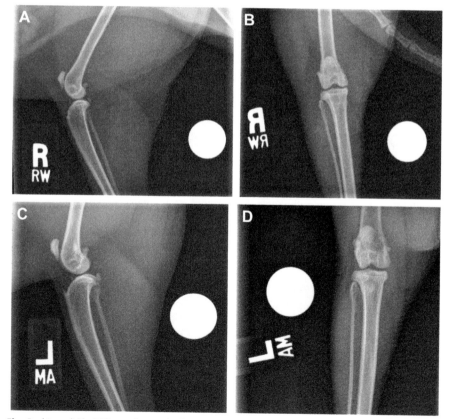

Fig. 2. (A and B): Stifle radiographs from a 9-year-old female spayed DSH demonstrating a patellar ligament enthesopathy and meniscal ossicle. (C and D): Stifle radiographs from a 12-year-old female spayed DSH demonstrating a mild medial meniscal ossification.

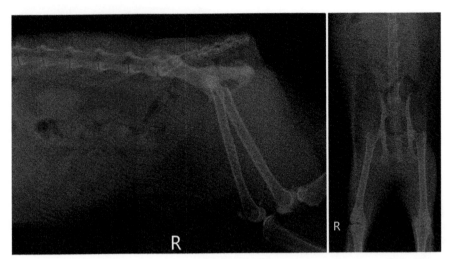

Fig. 3. Pelvic radiographs of a 14-year-old female spayed DSH demonstrating mild lumbosacral spondylosis deformans.

feasible for clinical use. Collar-mounted accelerometers can be used for activity monitoring and improvements in activity counts have been shown in cats with OA undergoing successful treatment.[13] Thermal and sensory threshold testing are demonstrated to be able to differentiate healthy limbs from those affected by OA.[14] Kinetic gait analysis, which is frequently used as a gold standard for objective lameness assessment in dogs, was not able to differentiate limbs affected by OA versus those free of disease, and therefore may not be useful in cats as an assessment or monitoring tool.[14]

INTEGRATIVE MANAGEMENT OF FELINE OSTEOARTHRITIS

In addition to causing pain and decreased mobility, feline OA can lead to behavioral problems such as aggression, house-soiling, altered social interactions, and loss of the human-animal bond.[15] All of these effects can contribute to QOL concerns and consideration of humane euthanasia. Multimodal intervention should be considered to alleviate clinical signs and slow progression of feline OA, often including analgesic medications, dietary modifications, nutraceuticals, environmental modifications, and physical rehabilitation. Regenerative medicine and acupuncture (AP) can also be considered, although research is lacking for feline OA.

Pharmacologic Management

Nonsteroidal anti-inflammatory drugs

Nonsteroidal anti-inflammatory drugs (NSAIDs) are often the first analgesic choice for OA pain across species. NSAIDs have been shown to improve activity and behavior in cats with chronic musculoskeletal diseases; however, there is less efficacy and safety data in cats compared with humans and dogs.[16] As of March 2021, only 2 NSAIDs, meloxicam and robenacoxib, were registered for long-term use ($\geq$7 days) in cats in Europe, and none was registered in the United States.[16,17] Clinical data for these NSAIDs are summarized in **Table 1**. The high prevalence of chronic kidney disease (CKD) among geriatric cats is one of the most common concerns for chronic NSAID use in feline OA. Clinicians must therefore weigh the potential risks versus benefits in felines with these concurrent diseases.

Table 1
Common analgesics for feline chronic pain

Medication	Dose	Notes	References
Meloxicam	Initial: 0.3 mg/kg SC once OR 0.1–0.2 mg/kg PO once Maintenance: 0.01–0.05 mg/kg PO q24–48h	Only labeled in the United States for cats as a single dose. Improved activity and ability to jump after 4–6 wk. Safe with stable CKD but monitor for new/worsening azotemia and proteinuria	6,15,16,18,20,22
Robenacoxib	SC: 2 mg/kg SC q24 h for a max of 3 d PO: 1–2.4 mg/kg PO q24 h × 6d for acute pain × 28d for OA	Well-tolerated, including cats with stable CKD Improvements in both objective and subjective outcome measures after 3–6 wk Effective in both acute and chronic pain conditions and demonstrates wide safety margin after short-term and long-term administration Pulsed therapy or titrate to lowest effective doses given every 2–3 d	16,17,19,23
Gabapentin	10 mg/kg PO q8–12 h	Most commonly prescribed medication for the treatment of chronic musculoskeletal pain in cats Improved activity, higher pain thresholds, and improved QOL Side effects: reduced activity, sedation, ataxia, weakness, muscle tremors	24–26
Tramadol	1–4 mg/kg PO q12 h	2mg/kg improved weight-bearing, mobility, comfort, and QOL Dose-dependent side effects: mydriasis, euphoria, dysphoria, sedation, hyporexia, diarrhea	Guedes et al,[27] 2018 & Monteiro et al,[28] 2017
Amantadine	3–5 mg/kg PO q24 h	Improved activity and QOL after 2–3 wk Side effects: self-limiting vomiting	Shipley et al,[29] 2021
Frunevetmab	1 - 2.8 mg/kg SC q3-4 wk	Blocks receptor-mediated signaling cascade induced by NGF Improved mobility in cats with OA in 6–8 wk Repeated dosing well-tolerated	Gruen [21] 2021

Clinics care points

For cats with concurrent OA and *stable* CKD.

- Use the lowest effective NSAID dose as part of a multimodal analgesic approach, pulsed therapy can be considered.[15,18,19]
- Maintenance of proper hydration is paramount.[20]
- Routine monitoring (recommended every 6 months) should be performed and the risks of chronic NSAID administration should be discussed with owners.[15]

Additional analgesics

Multimodal analgesia is becoming increasingly common for feline patients suffering from chronic pain conditions including OA. Common second-line oral analgesics include gabapentin, tramadol, and amantadine. More recently, Frunevetmab, an injectable felinized monoclonal antibody that binds to nerve growth factor (NGF), has been approved in the United States for use in cats with OA.[21] **Table 1** summarizes current research and recommendations for these analgesics in feline OA. Other oral analgesics, such as buprenorphine, amitriptyline, and grapiprant, lack clinical evidence for chronic feline pain and, therefore, will not be discussed.

Regenerative Medicine

There are only 2 studies evaluating the properties of platelet-rich plasma (PRP) products using feline blood. One study demonstrated a decrease in red and white blood cell (RBC and WBC) concentrations for 2 commercial systems but neither system showed adequate platelet concentrations.[30] Another study, using a different commercial system, reported significantly increased platelet concentrations and decreased RBC and WBC concentrations.[31] Currently, there are no prospective clinical trials investigating the efficacy of PRP for feline OA but it could be a promising therapeutic option based on human, equine, and canine literature. Similarly, no prospective studies have evaluated the use of stem cells in feline OA, although studies have shown promise for stem cell use in other chronic inflammatory feline conditions, such as inflammatory bowel disease and gingivostomatitis.[32] More feline studies are indicated to evaluate the clinical efficacy and safety of regenerative medical techniques in feline OA.

Dietary Considerations

Several studies have detected significant, positive associations between cats being overweight and having musculoskeletal conditions, including OA.[33] These findings are consistent with those in humans and dogs, for which being overweight is a well-known risk factor for OA and even modest weight loss, 6.1% body weight or more, has been demonstrated to significantly lower clinical signs associated with OA.[33,34] The contribution of adipose tissue to an inflammatory state through elevation of proinflammatory adipokines has been established in humans, and feline research also shows a correlation between adiposity and adipokine concentration.[33,35] Although further research is indicated to elucidate the relationship between overweight condition and feline OA, given the current evidence, weight loss should be a primary goal for overweight cats with concurrent OA.[36] Although a thorough discussion on feline weight loss is outside the scope of this article, **Table 2** summarizes dietary strategies to consider for cats with OA, including weight loss if indicated. In addition to caloric restriction, choosing a diet that supports the maintenance of lean body mass (LBM) and a feeding strategy to increase physical activity are advantageous weight-loss strategies.[35,37] Therapeutic diets supplemented with nutraceuticals or herbals will be discussed in the next section.

Table 2
Dietary strategies for feline osteoarthritis

Goal	Dietary Strategy

Weight loss
    Indicated for cats with a body
    condition score of 6+/9
    (overweight or obese)
	Restricted feeding of a moderate-high protein,
	    high-fiber diet formulated for weight loss:[37,40]
	Feed 80% of cat's current daily caloric intake
	    (often ~200 kcal/d)
	OR feed 80% of resting energy requirement for
	    ideal body weight
	Goal weight loss rate: 1.5% body weight/week
	Tips for success:[37]
	    Use a gram scale to measure meal portions
	    Allow 10% of daily calories from treats/pill
	        pockets/supplements
	    Feed cats in household separately
	    Divide daily diet into 2+ meals per day
	    Regular weight checks and caloric adjustment
	    Continue diet formulated for weight loss to
	        prevent rebound weight gain

Increase/maintain muscle mass
    Especially for sarcopenic or
    cachexic cats
	Provide adequate calories and dietary protein, especially
	    leucine (branched chain amino acid)[39]
	For sarcopenic, disease-free cats: 120–160g
	    protein/1000 kcal
	Consider addition of high-leucine protein sources (eg,
	    whey, egg white, low-fat cottage cheese, chicken
	    breast, soy)
	Manage concurrent diseases to minimize cachexia
	    (eg, CKD, cardiac disease, hyperthyroidism, cancer)[38,39]
	Provide adequate marine-sourced omega-3 fatty acids
	    and vitamin D, and consider an alkalinizing diet for
	    sarcopenic cats[39,41]
	0.4–1.5 g combined EPA and DHA/1000 kcal

Increase physical activity	Increase social interaction with humans surrounding
	    feeding and feeding frequency (2–4 meals/d)[42–44]
	Consider: puzzle feeders, feeding at varied elevations to
	    promote climbing[37]

Although young and middle-age domestic cats have a propensity for weight gain, middle-age and geriatric cats often lose weight and LBM concurrent with chronic disease processes (cachexia) or advancing age (sarcopenia).[37–39] This subset of cats with OA will require dietary intervention primarily to optimize maintenance or gain of LBM, in order to reduce muscle weakness and optimize mobility.[38] Incorporating feeding strategies to increase physical activity is advantageous in cats with both decreased LBM and OA, to promote regular, controlled exercise and muscle strengthening.[38]

Herbals and Supplements

There is a paucity of literature evaluating the use of herbals and supplements for the management of feline OA, with more robust research available in dogs and humans.[36,45] **Table 3** summarizes the current feline literature, inclusive of studies evaluating supplements, herbals, and supplemented therapeutic diets. There is growing evidence in feline OA for the use of omega-3 fatty acids (θ-3 FA), such as fish oil and green-lipped mussel (GLM) containing eicosapentaenoic acid (EPA) and docosahexaenoic acid (DHA), including high-quality trials evaluating objective outcome

Table 3
Evidence for herbals and supplements in feline osteoarthritis

Ref.[a]	n[b]	Study Design[c], Control (C)	Supplement[d]	Dose[e], Duration	OMs[f]	Outcomes[g] (vs C)	Adverse Events
Corbee et al,[47] 2013	24	RCT(crossover), C: corn oil (with fish smell)	ϴ-3 FA (Fish Oil)	1.8 g E + D/Mcal, 10 wk	CMI	Sign.: CMI (some items) NSD: CMI (some items)	Vomiting (4/24), dislike taste (3/24)
Lascelles et al,[46] 2010	43	RCT (parallel group), C: control diet	Test diet: ϴ-3 FA (Fish Oil and GLM), G + CS	1.9 g E + D/Mcal, 74 mg GLM/Mcal, 0.25 g G + CS/Mcal, 9 wk	CMI, AC, SOS	Sign.: AC, CMI (VAS) NSD: CMI (CSOM, QOL), SOS	Vomiting (1/43), dislike taste (1/43)
Corbee[48] 2022	26	RCT (crossover), C: placebo	SynopetCani-Syn (GLM, Curc, BLE)	3mL/d, 10 wk	CMI	Sign.: CMI (some items on HCPI) NSD: CMI (overall HCPI score)	Dislike taste (6/26)
Sul[49] 2014	31	RCT (crossover and parallel group) C: placebo and pos. control (meloxicam)	G + CS, Vit C, Zinc	250 mg G 175 mg CS 25 mg Vit C 15 mg Zinc, 2X/day X42 d followed by 1X/day X28 d	CMI SOS	NSD	Vomiting (1/31)

[a] Reference number.
[b] n, number of cats in trial.
[c] RCT, randomized controlled trial.
[d] BLE, blackcurrant leaf extract; CS, chondroitin sulfate; Curc, curcumin; G, glucosamine; Vit, vitamin.
[e] E + D, EPA + DHA; mcal, Megacalories.
[f] AC, activity count; CMI, clinical metrology instrument (client completed); SOS, subjective orthopedic score (veterinarian completed).
[g] CSOM, client-specific outcome measures; HCPI, helsinki chronic pain index; NSD, no significant difference in all or specified OM between groups; QOL, quality of life; Sign, statistically significant improvement in specified OM for the intervention group vs control; VAS, visual analog scale.

measures.[45–47] More evidences are needed to support the use of other herbals and supplements in feline OA.[45,48,49]

When recommending herbals and supplements, it is important to not only consider evidence of efficacy for a clinical indication but also evidence of bioavailability and safety, including independent laboratory testing of products for active ingredient concentrations and potential contaminants.[50–52] This information can be found in the primary literature, on product manufacturer websites (eg, a certificate of analysis), and in product reports from independent laboratories.[51] Veterinarians and consumers can also look for quality seals on products, such as the National Animal Supplement Council or ConsumerLab seal.

Although there are currently no studies evaluating the use of cannabidiol (CBD) for the management of feline OA, there are several studies describing pharmacokinetics and safety of CBD in cats, as well as evidence of efficacy of CBD for canine OA.[45,53,54] Feline CBD safety studies report overall tolerance of this herb, with a potential for mild side effects, such as hypersalivation, licking, vomiting and head-shaking.[53–55] Research evaluating the efficacy of CBD as part of the multimodal analgesic management feline OA is indicated.[45,53]

Clinics care points

- There is increasing evidence to support the use of fish oil for feline OA at a dose of 1.9 g combined EPA + DHA/Mcal (or 350–500 mg combined EPA + DHA per day for most cats). The authors recommend gradual introduction of fish oil starting with one-fourth to one-half the goal dose.
- More evidence is needed to support the use of other herbals and supplements in feline OA, such as CBD and GLM.
- Veterinarians must consider evidence of efficacy, bioavailability, and safety for herbals and supplements, including independent laboratory testing of products for active ingredient concentrations and potential contaminants.

Acupuncture

AP has been around for thousands of years as part of traditional Chinese medicine and is becoming more popular as an adjunct to Western medicine, especially for multimodal analgesia. Traditionally, AP has been used to restore balance or health to the body via local tissue stimulation and overall systemic effects.[56,57] Neurotransmitters (eg, serotonin, dopamine) and endogenous opioids are released in response to stimulation, contributing to analgesic, sedative, and neurostimulatory effects.[57] In addition, several studies have evaluated the physiologic effects of AP on OA, demonstrating reduced expression of inflammatory mediators and reduced cartilage matrix degeneration.[58,59]

A recent review reported 12 studies evaluating physiologic parameters and/or analgesic effects of AP in cats, as well as 1 study and 5 case reports/series evaluating AP for feline musculoskeletal conditions.[60] This review concluded that additional high-quality trials are indicated for further evaluation of AP efficacy in small animals.[60] In the authors' experience, many cats tolerate AP well as an adjunctive analgesic (**Fig. 4**). **Table 4** summarizes common AP techniques utilized for feline patients. The authors often begin with dry needle AP using acupoints along the back (Bladder meridian) and then introduce electroacupuncture. If traditional needling is not well tolerated, acupressure, laser AP, or aqua-AP can be used to stimulate points.

Physical Rehabilitation

Veterinary rehabilitation focuses on reducing pain, improving mobility, and returning animals to proper function. This is a growing field with many techniques used in

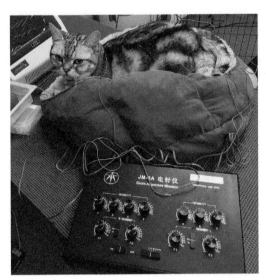

Fig. 4. A cat receiving electroacupuncture, an AP technique using electrical stimulation of needles placed in acupoints.

humans adapted for veterinary use. Currently, there are limited clinical studies in feline rehabilitation, with most recommendations translated from canine and human literature.

Manual therapies

Manual therapies should be relaxing and stress free for the most beneficial effects.[15,61] Some basic techniques include massage, passive movements, stretches, mobilization, manipulation, thermotherapy (heat), and cryotherapy (ice).[61] These techniques can be taught to owners, and can help to alleviate muscle pain, improve owner-pet interactions/bond, and improve QOL.[15,62]

Heat, massage, stretch, and passive ROM are generally well tolerated by cats in the authors' experience. We recommend performing these therapies in a quiet location where they are most comfortable (eg, away from other patients, on a bed or blanket). These therapies can help maintain joint health and improve muscle sensitivities.[56] Cryotherapy is often less tolerated but can be attempted for acute injuries or following exercise. Manipulative (chiropractic) therapies are minimally evidenced in small animals and adverse effects are of potential concern.[63] It has been recommended to consider low-velocity/low-impact methods in small animal geriatric patients if manipulative therapies are pursued.[63]

Table 4
Common techniques used to stimulate acupoints in cats

AP Technique	Description
Dry needle AP	Placement of small gauge needle into acupoints
Electroacupuncture	Electric leads applied to needles placed into acupoints
Laser AP	Application of therapeutic laser directly to an acupoint
Aqua-AP	Injection of a sterile liquid into an acupoint (eg, vitamin B12)
Acupressure	Manual pressure at an acupoint

Modalities

Laser therapy. To the authors' knowledge, no feline laser therapy studies for OA exist. However, human and canine OA studies demonstrate potential benefit, especially when applied at higher power densities (**Table 5**).[64–66] Laser therapy is generally well tolerated by cats because it is a relatively hands-off therapy delivered over a short time span (**Fig. 5**). Research is indicated to determine efficacy, safety, and optimize laser protocols for feline OA.

Therapeutic ultrasound. Therapeutic ultrasound is also well tolerated in feline patients and can be used for a variety of conditions (see **Table 5**). It is important to consider that cats have less dense soft tissues and smaller treatment areas than dogs; therefore, lower intensities should be used.[67] Ensure that all ultrasound gel is removed so large amounts are not ingested following therapy.

Electrical stimulation. Transcutaneous electrical nerve stimulation (TENS), similar to AP, provides symptomatic pain relief by exciting sensory nerves, which stimulate the pain gate mechanism and the release of endogenous opioids (see **Table 5**).[61] Electrodes can be placed over affected joints, spinal segments innervating affected joints, and/or over myofascial trigger or AP points. Neuromuscular electrical stimulation (NMES) is used to stimulate motor nerves and is useful in cats that cannot control voluntary movement or that cannot tolerate active exercise.[68] Electrical pads are optimally placed to elicit muscle contractions, contributing to muscle strengthening (see **Table 5**). These modalities may be well tolerated by cats but do require the use of gel and/or clipping of the haircoat, which may not be desirable. In addition, these can be uncomfortable or elicit a foreign sensation, so it is best to start slow and use low-intensity settings. An advantage of these modalities is they can be taught to owners and performed at home, which is both cost-effective and low-stress to the patient.

Pulsed electromagnetic field therapy. Pulsed electromagnetic field (PEMF) therapy can be used for acute and chronic injuries to improve cellular repair by increasing the local perfusion to the capillary blood flow.[68] Veterinary studies have demonstrated benefits of PEMF treatment of canine OA, with reduced clinical signs following a series

Table 5
Common modalities for feline osteoarthritis management

Modality	Indications	References
Laser therapy	Wound healing, pain management, anti-inflammatory, fractures, tendon/ligament injuries Improve pain, lameness/stiffness, and function in patients with OA	56,61,64–66,68
Therapeutic ultrasound	Restricted ROM, joint contracture, pain management, muscle spasm, remodeling of scar tissue, tendon/ligament injuries, enhance tissue repair, wound/fracture healing	56,61,67
TENS	Pain control, decrease muscle spasm, decrease edema	56,61,68
NMES	Muscle strengthening, decrease muscle atrophy, improve limb function	Millis [56] 2014 & Halkett [68] 2017
PEMF	Pain control, reduce inflammation/edema, tissue/wound healing May reduce pain and signs of OA	56,68,69

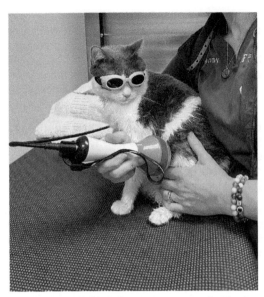

Fig. 5. A cat receiving laser therapy for pain management of stifle OA.

of treatments (9–20) of 18 to 60-minute duration.[69] This modality is typically delivered via a bed or small portable device and can be performed at home or during rehabilitation sessions. This treatment has no sensation and is well tolerated by felines. Devices can be placed in the cat's current bed or other frequented areas.

Therapeutic exercise
Therapeutic exercise, especially muscle strengthening, is one of the most important parts of the rehabilitation process for cats with OA and should be personalized to individual needs.[70] Exercise can be used to decrease pain, improve aerobic capacity, endurance, agility, coordination, balance, gait, movement patterning, postural stabilization, ROM, and strength.[61] Exercise can be divided into 4 main types including strengthening, flexibility, balance/proprioception, and endurance.[61] Feline rehabilitation poses a unique challenge; practitioners must understand the behaviors of cats and how to motivate them without causing stress. Cats can be motivated by having them follow a lure toy, laser pointer, food/treats, or by having them walk toward their carriers. Creativity is very helpful when motivating cats to perform these exercises in hospital and at home. Assistive devices or special equipment can be used to supplement exercises as needed. **Table 6 (Fig. 6)** discusses specific examples of therapeutic exercises commonly used for feline OA based on overall therapeutic goal.

Hydrotherapy
Underwater treadmill therapy and swimming can be well tolerated in cats with slow introduction, short sessions, and positive reinforcement **(Fig. 7)**.[67] The natural properties of water (eg, density, buoyancy, viscosity, resistance, hydrostatic pressure, surface tension) make water-based exercise one of the most useful forms of rehabilitation therapy by reducing the concussive effects of active exercise and improving limb mobility, strength, and joint ROM.[56,61] Hydrotherapy can also be used to relieve pain, reduce swelling and stiffness, aid in weight loss, and improve blood circulation.[57] If available, starting on a land treadmill may be beneficial to acclimate cats to the moving belt. If tolerated, transition to standing in water and then

Table 6
Common therapeutic exercises for feline osteoarthritis

Goal	Examples	References
Strengthening	Running (controlled), land treadmill, up/down inclines, leg/body weights, resistance bands, dancing (forwards/backwards), wheelbarrowing, hydrotherapy	56,61,68
Flexibility	Crawling under, over, or through objects, weaving, reaching, cookie stretches, cavalettis	Sharp [61] 2012 & Halkett [68] 2017
Balance/proprioception	Balance on uneven surface (eg, wobble board, rocker board, peanut), walking over objects (cavalettis) **(Fig. 7)**, walking in circles, figure eights, weaving, walking over different textured surfaces, weight shifting, rhythmic stabilization	Sharp [61] 2012 & Halkett [68] 2017
Endurance	Hydrotherapy or active exercise >15 min several times a week	Sharp [61] 2012

slowly increase the speed of the treadmill so the patient is at a slow comfortable walk. The authors' recommend staging hydrotherapy introduction in this way, gradually increasing the duration of therapy and discontinuing therapy if the patient seems stressed.

Environmental Considerations

OA may cause impaired mobility and activity due to chronic pain. Cats should have easy access to food, water, litter boxes, areas to hide, and resting spaces. Litter boxes

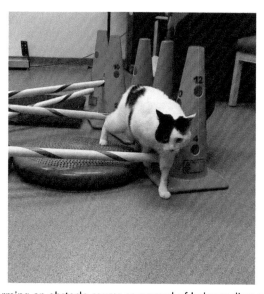

Fig. 6. A cat performing an obstacle course composed of balance discs and cavaletti poles.

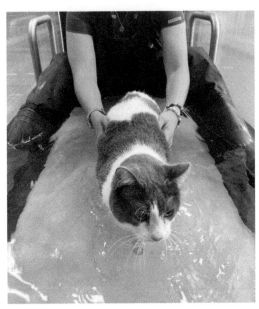

Fig. 7. A cat walking on the underwater treadmill for weight loss and hindlimb strengthening.

with lower edges may be easier to step into.[15,62] Enclosed boxes may assist owners in dealing with abnormal elimination habits, such as cats eliminating while standing due to a reluctance to posture.[15] Access to heights, such as furniture and windows, is important, and mobility-impaired cats may have a more difficult time accessing these areas.[15,62] Movement of furniture to provide "stepped" access, pet stairs, or ramps can be used to provide easier access to preferred resting areas.[15,62]

A more complex home environment will also encourage more movement, which is beneficial in maintaining joint health, muscle mass, promoting an ideal body condition, and providing mental stimulation.[15,22,62] Walking over uneven surfaces, providing scratching posts, cat towers, toys, and hiding food will encourage natural behaviors such as foraging, hunting, and playing.[15,62] Regular periods of play with laser pointers, toys, and catnip will also increase exercise levels.[15,62]

SUMMARY

Management of feline OA involves unique challenges in the timely identification of the disease due to subtle or vague clinical signs and in formulation of a treatment plan. Few analgesic medications are approved for long-term use in cats for the management of OA; care must be taken when selecting analgesic medications in regards to the presence of concurrent disease and consideration of possible side effects. Dietary considerations include weight loss for overweight cats, appropriate protein intake to maintain LBM, and feeding strategies to maintain light activity. A growing number of nutraceuticals are marketed for feline OA with limited evidence of bioavailability, efficacy, or safety; the greatest evidence currently exists for beneficial effects of marine-sourced θ-3 FAs. Physical rehabilitation incorporates manual therapies, therapeutic modalities, and exercise to provide adjunctive pain relief, maximize joint ROM, and strengthen muscles to support mobility; feline rehabilitation may be initially limited by patient tolerance but often can be accomplished with patience and creativity in planning. Environmental modifications are recommended to reduce functional impairments of OA by providing easier access to necessities (food, water, litterbox) and resting places. Additional research is needed in the roles of AP and regenerative medicine for the management of feline OA. With numerous treatment options available, a multimodal approach allows the practitioner and cat owner to find the best treatment plan to maximize QOL.

DISCLOSURE

The authors have nothing to disclose.

DECLARATION OF INTERESTS

The authors have no conflict of interest to disclose.

REFERENCES

1. Kimura T, Kimura S, Okada J, et al. Retrospective radiographic study of degenerative joint disease in cats: prevalence based on orthogonal radiographs. Front Vet Sci 2020;7:138.
2. Clarke SP, Mellor D, Clements DN, et al. Prevalence of radiographic signs of degenerative joint disease in a hospital population of cats. Vet Rec 2005;157(25):793–9.
3. Godfrey DR. Osteoarthritis in cats: a retrospective radiological study. J Small Anim Pract 2005;46(9):425–9.
4. Hardie EM, Roe SC, Martin FR. Radiographic evidence of degenerative joint disease in geriatric cats: 100 cases (1994-1997). J Am Vet Med Assoc 2002;220(5): 628–32.
5. Lascelles BDX, Henry JB III, Brown J, et al. Cross-sectional study of the prevalence of radiographic degenerative joint disease in domesticated cats. Vet Surg 2010;39(5):535–44.
6. Clarke SP, Bennett D. Feline osteoarthritis: a prospective study of 28 cases. J Small Anim Pract 2006;47(8):439–45.
7. Kranenburg HC, Meij BP, van Hofwegen EML, et al. Prevalence of spondylosis deformans in the feline spine and correlation with owner-perceived behavioral changes. Vet Comp Orthop Traumatol 2012;25(3):217–23.
8. Lascelles BDX, Dong YH, Marcellin-Little DJ, et al. Relationship of orthopedic examination, goniometric measurements, and radiographic signs of degenerative joint disease in cats. BMC Vet Res 2012;8:10.
9. Tsai CY, Chang YP. Assessment of the cutaneous trunci muscle reflex in healthy cats: comparison of results acquired by clinicians and cat owners. J Fel Med Surg 2022;24(8):e163–7.
10. Freire M, Robertson I, Bondell HD, et al. Radiographic evaluation of feline appendicular degenerative joint disease vs. macroscopic appearance of articular cartilage. Vet Radiol Ultrasound 2011;52(3):239–47.
11. Benito J, Depuy V, Hardie E, et al. Reliability and discriminatory testing of a client-based metrology instrument, feline musculoskeletal pain index (FMPI) for the evaluation of degenerative joint disease-associated pain in cats. Vet J 2013; 196(3):368–73.
12. Benito J, Hansen B, Depuy V, et al. Feline musculoskeletal pain index: responsiveness and testing of criterion validity. J Vet Intern Med 2013;27(3):474–82.

13. Lascelles BDX, Bernie HD, Roe S, et al. Evaluation of client-specific outcome measures and activity monitoring to measure pain relief in cats with osteoarthritis. J Vet Intern Med 2007;21(3):410–6.

14. Addison ES, Clements DN. Repeatability of quantitative sensory testing in healthy cats in a clinical setting with comparison to cats with osteoarthritis. J Feline Med Surg 2017;19(12):1274–82.

15. Perry K. Feline hip dysplasia: a challenge to recognize and treat. J Feline Med Surg 2016;18(3):203–18.

16. King JN, Seewald W, Forster S, et al. Clinical safety of robenacoxib in cats with chronic musculoskeletal disease. J Vet Intern Med 2021;35(5):2384–94.

17. Lees P, Toutain PL, Elliott J, et al. Pharmacology, safety, efficacy and clinical uses of the COX-2 inhibitor robenacoxib. J Vet Pharmacol Ther 2022;45(4):325–51.

18. Gowan RA, Lingard AE, Johnston L, et al. Retrospective case-control study of the effects of long-term dosing with meloxicam on renal function in aged cats with degenerative joint disease. J Feline Med Surg 2011;13(10):752–61.

19. King JN, King S, Budsberg SC, et al. Clinical safety of robenacoxib in feline osteoarthritis: results of a randomized, blinded, placebo-controlled clinical trial. J Feline Med Surg 2016;18(8):632–42.

20. KuKanich K, George C, Roush JK, et al. Effects of low-dose meloxicam in cats with chronic kidney disease. J Feline Med Surg 2021;23(2):138–48.

21. Gruen ME, Myers JAE, Lascelles BDX. Efficacy and safety of an anti-nerve growth factor antibody (frunevetmab) for the treatment of degenerative joint disease-associated chronic pain in cats: a multi-site pilot field study. Front Vet Sci 2021; 8:610028.

22. Bennett D, Affrin S, Johnston P. Osteoarthritis in the cat: 2. how should it be managed and treated? J Feline Med Surg 2012;14(1):76–84.

23. Adrian D, King JN, Parrish RS, et al. Robenacoxib shows efficacy for the treatment of chronic degenerative joint disease-associated pain in cats: a randomized and blinded pilot clinical trial. Sci Rep 2021;11(1):7721.

24. Guedes AGP, Meadows JM, Pypendop BH, et al. Assessment of the effects of gabapentin on activity levels and owner-perceived mobility impairment and quality of life in osteoarthritic geriatric cats. J Am Vet Med Assoc 2018;253(5):579–85.

25. Adrian D, Papich MG, Baynes R, et al. The pharmacokinetics of gabapentin in cats. J Vet Intern Med 2018;32(6):1996–2002.

26. Klinck MP, Monteiro BP, Lussier B, et al. Refinement of the Montreal Instrument for Cat Arthritis Testing, for Use by Veterinarians: detection of naturally occurring osteoarthritis in laboratory cats. J Feline Med Surg 2018;20(8):728–40.

27. Guedes AGP, Meadows JM, Pypendop BH, et al. Evaluation of tramadol for treatment of osteoarthritis in geriatric cats. J Am Vet Med Assoc 2018;252(5):565–71.

28. Monteiro BP, Klinck MP, Moreau M, et al. Analgesic efficacy of tramadol in cats with naturally occurring osteoarthritis. PLoS One 2017;12(4):e0175565.

29. Shipley H, Flynn K, Tucker L, et al. Owner evaluation of quality of life and mobility in osteoarthritic cats treated with amantadine or placebo. J Feline Med Surg 2021;23(6):568–74.

30. Ferrari JT, Schwartz P. Prospective evaluation of feline sourced platelet-rich plasma using centrifuge-based systems. Front Vet Sci 2020 Jun;7:322.

31. Chun N, Canapp S, Carr BJ, et al. Validation and characterization of platelet-rich plasma in the feline: a prospective analysis. Front Vet Sci 2020;7:512.

32. Webb TL. Stem cell therapy and cats: what do we know at this time? Vet Clin North Am Small Anim Pract 2020;50(5):955–71.

33. Teng KT, McGreevy PD, Toribio JL, et al. Strong associations of nine-point body condition scoring with survival and lifespan in cats. J Feline Med Surg 2018; 20(12):1110–8.
34. Marshall WG, Hazewinkel HA, Mullen D, et al. The effect of weight loss on lameness in obese dogs with osteoarthritis. Vet Res Commun 2010;34(3):241–53.
35. Frye CW, Shmalberg JW, Wakshlag JJ. Obesity, exercise and orthopedic disease. Vet Clin North Am Small Anim Pract 2016;46(5):831–41.
36. Johnson KA, Lee AH, Swanson KS. Nutrition and nutraceuticals in the changing management of osteoarthritis for dogs and cats. J Am Vet Med Assoc 2020; 256(12):1335–41.
37. German AJ. Obesity prevention and weight maintenance after loss. Vet Clin North Am Small Anim Pract 2016;46(5):913–29.
38. Freeman LM. Cachexia and sarcopenia: emerging syndromes of importance in dogs and cats. J Vet Intern Med 2012;26(1):3–17.
39. Saker KE. Nutritional concerns for cancer, cachexia, frailty, and sarcopenia in canine and feline pets. Vet Clin North Am Small Anim Pract 2021;51(3):729–44.
40. Pallotto MR, de Godoy MRC, Holscher HD, et al. Effects of weight loss with a moderate-protein, high-fiber diet on body composition, voluntary physical activity, and fecal microbiota of obese cats. Am J Vet Res 2018;79(2):181–90.
41. Hall JA, Jackson MI, Farace G, et al. Influence of dietary ingredients on lean body percent, uremic toxin concentrations, and kidney function in senior-adult cats. Metabolites 2019;9(10):238.
42. de Godoy MR, Shoveller AK. Overweight adult cats have significantly lower voluntary physical activity than adult lean cats. J Feline Med Surg 2017;19(12): 1267–73.
43. de Godoy MR, Ochi K, de Oliveira Mateus LF, et al. Feeding frequency, but not dietary water content, affects voluntary physical activity in young lean adult female cats. J Anim Sci 2015;93(5):2597–601.
44. Deng P, Grant RW, Swanson KS. Physical activity level of adult cats with varied feeding frequency. Br J Nutr 2011;106(S1):S166–9.
45. Barbeau-Grégoire M, Otis C, Cournoyer A, et al. 2022 systematic review and meta-analysis of enriched therapeutic diets and nutraceuticals in canine and feline osteoarthritis. Int J Mol Sci 2022;23(18):10384.
46. Lascelles BDX, DePuy V, Thomson A, et al. Evaluation of a therapeutic diet for feline degenerative joint disease. J Vet Intern Med 2010;24(3):487–95.
47. Corbee RJ, Barnier MMC, van de Lest CHA, et al. The effect of dietary long-chain omega-3 fatty acid supplementation on owner's perception of behaviour and locomotion in cats with naturally occurring osteoarthritis. J Anim Physiol Anim Nutr 2013;97(5):846–53.
48. Corbee RJ. The efficacy of a nutritional supplement containing green-lipped mussel, curcumin and blackcurrant leaf extract in dogs and cats with osteoarthritis. Vet Med Sci 2022;8(3):1025–35.
49. Sul RM, Chase D, Parkin T, et al. Comparison of meloxicam and a glucosamine-chondroitin supplement in management of feline osteoarthritis. A double-blind randomised, placebo-controlled, prospective trial. Vet Comp Orthop Traumatol 2014;27(1):20–6.
50. Lenox CE, Bauer JE. Potential adverse effects of omega-3 fatty acids in dogs and cats. J Vet Intern Med 2013;27(2):217–26.
51. Wakshlag JJ, Cital S, Eaton SJ, et al. Cannabinoid, terpene, and heavy metal analysis of 29 over-the-counter commercial veterinary hemp supplements. Vet Med 2020;11:45–55.

52. Miscioscia E, Shmalberg J, Scott KC. Measurement of 3-acetyl-11-keto-beta-boswellic acid and 11-keto-beta-boswellic acid in Boswellia serrata supplements administered to dogs. BMC Vet Res 2019;15(1):270.

53. Yu CHJ, Rupasinghe HPV. Cannabidiol-based natural health products for companion animals: Recent advances in the management of anxiety, pain, and inflammation. Res Vet Sci 2021;140:38–46.

54. Wang T, Zakharov A, Gomez B, et al. Serum cannabinoid 24 h and 1 week steady state pharmacokinetic assessment in cats using a CBD/CBDA rich hemp paste. Front Vet Sci 2022;9:895368.

55. Deabold KA, Schwark WS, Wolf L, et al. Single-dose pharmacokinetics and preliminary safety assessment with use of CBD-rich hemp nutraceutical in healthy dogs and cats. Animals 2019;9(10):832.

56. Millis DL, Levine D. Canine rehabilitation and physical therapy. 2nd edition. Philadelphia, PA: Elsevier Saunders; 2014.

57. Romano L, Halkett EVC. Rehabilitation of the feline patient: acupuncture and hydrotherapy as part of a multidisciplinary team approach. Vet Nurse 2018;9(1): 26–31.

58. Zhang Y, Bao F, Wang Y, et al. Influence of acupuncture in treatment of knee osteoarthritis and cartilage repairing. Am J Transl Res 2016;8(9):3995–4002.

59. Wang DH, Bao F, Wu Z, et al. Influence of acupuncture on IL-1beta and TNF-alpha expression in the cartilage of rats with knee arthritis. Zongguo Gu Shang 2011;24(9):775–8.

60. Rose WJ, Sargeant JM, Hanna WJB, et al. A scoping review of the evidence for efficacy of acupuncture in companion animals. Anim Health Res Rev 2017;18(2): 177–85.

61. Sharp B. Feline physiotherapy and rehabilitation: 1. principles and potential. J Feline Med Surg 2012;14(9):622–32.

62. Lascelles BDX, Robertson SA. DJD-associated pain in cats: what can we do to promote patient comfort? J Feline Med Surg 2010;12(3):200–12.

63. Kidd JR. Alternative medicines for the geriatric veterinary patient. Vet Clin North Am Small Anim Pract 2012;42(4):809–22, viii.

64. Looney AL, Huntingford JL, Blaeser LL, et al. A randomized blind placebo-controlled trial investigating the effects of photobiomodulation therapy (PBMT) on canine elbow osteoarthritis. Can Vet J 2018;59(9):959–66.

65. Barale L, Monticelli P, Raviola M, et al. Preliminary clinical experience of low-level laser therapy for the treatment of canine osteoarthritis-associated pain: A retrospective investigation on 17 dogs. Open Vet J 2020;10(1):116–9.

66. Song HJ, Seo HJ, Kim D. Effectiveness of high-intensity laser therapy in the management of patients with knee osteoarthritis: A systematic review and meta-analysis of randomized controlled trials. J Back Musculoskelet Rehabil 2020; 33(6):875–84.

67. Drum MG, Bockstahler B, Levine D, et al. Feline Rehabilitation. Vet Clin North Am Small Anim Pract 2015;45(1):185–201.

68. Halkett EVC, Romano L. Rehabilitation of the feline patient: physiotherapy treatment as part of a multidisciplinary team approach. Vet Nurse 2017;8(10):548–52.

69. Gaynor JS, Hagberg S, Gurfein BT. Veterinary applications of pulsed electromagnetic field therapy. Res Vet Sci 2018;119:1–8.

70. Herzog W, Longino D, Clark A. The role of muscles in joint adaptation and degeneration. Langenbeck's Arch Surg 2003;388(5):305–15.

Use of Rehabilitation Therapy in Palliative Care Patients

Jeret Benson, DVM, MS[a], Lindsey Fry, DVM, DACVSMR[b],
Jessica Rychel, DVM, DACVSMR[b],*

KEYWORDS

- Palliative care • Palliative rehabilitation • Hospice • Rehabilitation • Geriatric
- Disablement model • Function-targeted treatment

KEY POINTS

- Palliative rehabilitation can reduce caregiver burden and enhance professional satisfaction for the rehabilitation practitioner.
- Applying the disablement model can aid in the identification of treatment targets for palliative care patients and guide intervention selection.
- Functional-targeted treatment employs all available pharmacologic interventions and rehabilitation modalities to achieve appropriate goals for the patient and family.
- Treatments should not be withheld due to lack of diagnostics but selected with careful weighting of risk and benefit for the individual patient.

INTRODUCTION AND BACKGROUND
Defining Palliative Rehabilitation

Palliative care is the interdisciplinary, medical caregiving approach aimed at optimizing the quality of life and managing pain, without attempting to cure the underlying disease. Commonly, the terminology of palliative care is linked explicitly with hospice care, though hospice care should be considered a separate, though related, entity. Palliative care is something that rehabilitation practitioners do very well, as many patients begin a palliative care journey as soon as they incur a significant orthopedic or neurologic diagnosis as a middle-aged, or even young, patient. Such examples of long-term palliative care cases include a cat with early renal disease, a young dog diagnosed with early osteoarthritis, or a patient with geriatric-onset laryngeal paralysis

[a] Doctor of Veterinary Medicine, Red Sage Integrative Veterinary Partners, 1006 Luke Street, Fort Collins, CO 80524, USA; [b] Doctor of Veterinary Medicine and Diplomate of the American College of Veterinary, Sports Medicine and Rehabilitation, 1006 Luke Street, Fort Collins, CO 80524, USA
* Corresponding author.
E-mail address: jessrychel@redsagevets.com

Vet Clin Small Anim 53 (2023) 897–919
https://doi.org/10.1016/j.cvsm.2023.02.016
0195-5616/23/© 2023 Elsevier Inc. All rights reserved.

Table 1
Definition of a palliative care patient[1]

Qualifications	Examples
Diagnosed with a terminal disease	Metastatic cancer Renal failure Liver failure Advanced cardiovascular disease Pulmonary fibrosis Necrotizing meningoencephalitis Degenerative myelopathy
Chronic progressive disease	Cancer Congestive heart failure Renal insufficiency Osteoarthritis Lumbosacral stenosis Cervical spondylomyelopathy
Disability affecting mobility	Intervertebral disk disease Cruciate disease Dysplasia—hip, elbow, other
Geriatric disease	Geriatric onset of laryngeal paralysis and peripheral neuropathy (GOLPP) Cognitive dysfunction
Wasting and Sarcopenia	Loss of body condition and/or muscle mass in the absence of concurrent disease
Failure to thrive	Unknown diagnosis but loss of appetite, mobility, and interactivity lead to declining quality of life

polyneuropathy (**Table 1**). Helping to address the discomfort and disability of a chronic disease is well-suited to the gentle yet productive techniques and modalities that rehabilitation offers. In this article, you will find descriptions of those techniques with specific attention to those aspects helpful to patients more advanced in their palliative care journey and even those entering the realm of hospice care.

Cheville and colleagues define palliative rehabilitation based on these concepts in human patients with a terminal cancer diagnosis, *Palliative rehabilitation is function-directed care delivered in partnership with other disciplines and aligned with the values of patients who have serious and often incurable illnesses in contexts marked by intense and dynamic symptoms, psychological stress, and medical morbidity, to realize potentially time-limited goal.* [2] This definition transfers well to our veterinary palliative care patients and widens the scope of diagnosis and treatment goals.

Disablement Model and Functional-Targeted Treatment

The disablement model offers a way to approach medical conditions that accounts for an individual patient and their family's needs. It is a scaffolding to assess patients with a disability (injury or illness) based not only on their disease pathology, but how their quality of life and activities of daily living have been impacted. The model was developed by sociologist Saad Nagi in 1965 and has been built upon since that time in many human health care arenas, providing more ease in communication about case management.[3,4] The primary diagnosis, referred to as an active injury or illness, leads to a cascade of impacts on various levels, each individual to a given patient. This helps strategically explain why the experience and management of a similar diagnosis can vary widely between patients, as demonstrated in a comparative example within **Table 2**.

Table 2
Disablement model applied to veterinary patients

	Cellular Level		Patient #1 10 yo FS Standard Poodle IVDD- T3-L3 Myelopathy	Patient #2 7 yo MN Dachshund IVDD- T3-L3 Myelopathy
Active Pathology		Pathologic diagnosis, physiologic derangement		
Impairment	Body systems	Mobility (ie- ROM, flexibility), Muscle Function (Engagement, strength, muscle mass) Pain	• Pelvic limb paresis • Loss of urinary and fecal continence • Loss of muscle mass in the pelvic limbs • Unable to rise on her own	• Pelvic limb paresis, weakly ambulatory • Loss of muscle mass in the pelvic limbs • Significant pain at the TL junction
Functional limitations	Whole patients	Activities of daily living	• Is dependent on diapers • Cannot go outside without assistance to urinate and defecate • Cannot follow owners from room to room	• Hard to pick him up without pain, yelping and crying out frequently • Sometimes experiences incontinence due to level of pain with handling
Disability	Role in Family/Society	Jobs, Relationships, Human– Animal Bond	• Less interactive and tends to get lonely and frustrated, barking and becoming agitated • Loss of independence for elimination • Can no longer participate in agility and rally, a previous love of patient and client	• Used to be frequently carried by the owner and sit in her lap—cannot do this with the current level of back pain. She would be glad to carry him and hold him again • Hiding in his crate, seems to be scared and less interactive • Has snapped at the owner, directly impacting the human–animal bond between them

Clients tend to recognize disabilities and functional limitations in their pets and find them to be motivators for seeking care and intervention. Many pet owners receive their pet's diagnosis of active pathology and possible treatment options in a short period. That leaves them to make decisions on their own, including whether they wish to pursue curative treatment, palliative or hospice care. The client may have little understanding of the active disease process, but see changes in the function and day-to-day quality of life of their pet. This is also often how they will assess response to interventions. This is different from the provider perspective, where only a glimpse of their overall life is seen and traditionally the focus is on determining active pathology and curative treatment options. Understanding additional limitations and levels of disease allow for "function-directed" treatments and assessments. Communication about client perceptions of the pet's functional limitations and disability can bridge the gap between active pathology and disability, making planning easier and more successful.[5]

As rehab practitioners build trust with the patient, and get to know the client, they can slowly peel back layers of the disability to determine function-targeted goals most appropriate to that patient and family, **Table 3**. Clear goals, that the client has had a voice in creating, allow for more relevant outcome measurements as the rehab program progresses. If an intervention does not address these goals, even if it addresses a practitioner's goal, it may not be considered successful for the patient. This approach requires consistent re-evaluation of goals and interventions to meet these needs, as well as an ongoing partnership between client and practitioner.

It is beneficial to have a few clearly defined outcome measures to track progress. Frye *and colleagues* tackled this topic in geriatric patients, by suggesting the use of a Canine Geriatric Functional Score.[6] This score assesses strength, endurance, and balance/spatial awareness with a short series of testing. This offers a shift from strictly objective outcomes to functional outcome assessment which is more applicable when using a function-targeted treatment plan. Novel thinking in regard to tracking patient disablement, function, and mobility will help guide practitioners in their pursuit of function-targeted goals for palliative care patients.

Table 3
Determining disability to help establish function-targeted goals

Case #1	Case #2	Case #3
A 12-year-old female spayed Labrador with hip dysplasia and osteoarthritis (pathology) has weakness in her hind limbs and reluctance to jump (impairments). This causes difficulty in getting in and out of the car, onto the bed, and going on hikes (functional limitations), is not able to sleep with her owners and participate in outdoor activities (disability).	A 10-year-old male DSH with renal disease and hyperthyroidism and osteoarthritis (pathology) has significant cachexia and weakness (impairments). He cannot climb stairs or get into his cat tree where he prefers to sleep (functional limitations). He is more stressed without being able to get to higher locations and is hiding more which means less interaction with his family (disability).	A 14-yo-female spayed Cattle dog has no specific diagnoses (pathology), but her sight, hearing have diminished significantly in recent months and she seems confused (impairments). Gradually she stops interacting with the other dog in the house and is reluctant to go outside and will have accidents in the house causing frustration for her family (disability).

Caregiver Burden in the Palliative Care Setting

Caregiver burden is a newly explored topic in veterinary medicine defined as the emotional and physical stress experienced by the pet owner while caring for a pet with a chronic disease. There are many factors associated with caregiver burden including but not limited to, financial strain, time constraints, physical toll, and emotional toll.[7,8] In human medicine, caregiver burden has been associated with increased levels of daytime cortisol, anxiety, and depression.[8–10] Current research indicates that, although caregiver burden is multifactorial some common themes cause worsening stress, which include the patient's symptom severity, the time and number of tasks associated with caregiving, and the longer duration of caregiving during the disease/illness.[7] It should also be noted that clients stressed with caregiver burden can create undue stress on veterinary teams, including more non-billable veterinary contacts and repeat visits with higher levels of frustration and fear.[7] This has led veterinary professionals to feel they are providing futile care, contributing to burnout, and compassion fatigue in the field.[11]

Thankfully, rehabilitation can help to decrease the incidence of that burden for clients and the veterinary team caring for the patient. When palliative care patients are seen frequently for rehabilitation services, the owners are provided with tools for managing pain, evaluating suffering, enhancing mobility, and a variety of other educational tools that reduce their stress and enhance their confidence in caregiving. This also reduces non-billable contacts with the pet's veterinary team, including primary care veterinarian professionals, specialists, and the rehab practitioner, while reducing stress for those providers as well.

Another challenging topic that contributes to caregiver burden is the pursuit of diagnostic testing. Some families of palliative care patients are interested in maximizing quality of life while minimizing invasive and taxing tests and procedures. This should lift the burden for clinicians and rehab practitioners to pursue extensive diagnostic testing in the palliative care setting. Although for some conditions, understanding the exact etiology of the underlying problem is helpful, the initiation of rehabilitation for a palliative care patient should never be delayed due to lack of diagnostic testing.

CURRENT EVIDENCE AND RECOMMENDATIONS

As rehabilitation practitioners, we have access to a large toolbox of modalities and interventions that allow for individualized treatment plans. By using the disablement model for a patient, treatments can be selected based on all the regions of the model. A clear understanding of the indications, benefits, and also risks of intervention provides the foundation for creating effective and customized management plans.

Pharmacologic Management

Pain management is foundational in palliative care management plans and is frequently the primary goal of both pet owners and practitioners. Pain advances in these complex patients to become more maladaptive, so practitioners must manage both the primary pain issue and secondary maladaptive pain.[12] Most palliative care patients are on many medications, have one or more complicating comorbidities, and medicating them becomes more challenging with changes in appetite and caregiver fatigue. Being versatile and adaptive in pain management approaches for palliative care is critical for success. Understanding indications, mechanisms of action, potential risks, side effects, and appropriate monitoring, for multiple pain medications will help a rehabilitation practitioner choose from the wide variety of options available.

Risk-benefit analysis is important in these patients, especially when considering their timeline and level of pain. Often risks become less worrisome when the benefits are compelling for a palliative care patient.

There is an additional article dedicated to pain management for rehab patients, so the focus in **Table 4** will be analgesic options with a special focus on palliative care patients. Many of these medications are called "co-analgesics," and are considered when there is breakthrough pain in patients already on a good pain management plan, or in those whose pain is inadequately managed. Often these are used in combination and adjusted as needed or as symptoms change. This chart is meant as a guideline for choosing additional pain management options in palliative care patients with consideration of their indication and contraindications.

Rehabilitation Modalities for Palliative Care

Rehabilitation modalities often offer compelling additions to a palliative care plan, as they tend to be non-invasive while they have a high potential to improve comfort, mobility, and quality of life. Additionally, they can be used to tailor a treatment plan to the disablement of the pet and offer the practitioner and family the opportunity for frequent re-evaluation and adjustment in the patient's plan. See **Table 5** for details about some of the pros and cons of the individual modalities frequently used in the palliative care setting. Finally, **Table 6** references joint injections that can be used for patients with joint pain or lumbosacral disease and can be a helpful adjunct to any palliative care rehabilitation plan.

Pulsed Electromagnetic Field Therapy

Pulsed electromagnetic field therapy (PEMF) has grown in popularity and accessibility in veterinary rehabilitation medicine over the past decade and offers a compelling non-invasive therapy for the management of wound healing, bone healing, neurologic recovery, swelling and edema reduction, and pain management. A variety of veterinary-specific and human devices, including loops, mats, beds, and patches with embedded PEMF devices are available for clients to purchase for their pets. PEMF affects numerous cellular functions, though there are a few important mechanisms of action that apply directly to its use in the palliative care rehabilitation setting. PEMF exposure alters calcium release and binding with calmodulin which can impact inflammation, regional immune function, and pain signaling transduction. PEMF causes downregulation of inflammatory mediators like interleukin-6 (IL-6) and tumor necrosis factor (TNF)-alpha, which can contribute to pain, local inflammation, and tissue degradation in palliative care patients.[34]

Palliative care for geriatric or debilitated patients often includes wound care, which can contribute to loss of quality of life as well as exposure of veterinary team and client to chronic wound infections. PEMF has shown significant promise in the management and healing of wounds, even when chronic in nature. PEMF enhances angiogenesis, fibroblast migration, and inflammatory modulation, thereby, encouraging wound contraction and more rapid healing.[34,35] PEMF is also beneficial in osteoarthritis and neurologic injury, both of which are common comorbidities for patients in the palliative care setting. It is known that bony turnover, osteoblast activity and chondroblast health can be positively impacted by utilizing PEMF therapy, in addition to modulation in the metalloproteinase activity that naturally occurs in osteoarthritis patients.[36] Osteoarthritis patients (and owners) report improved quality of life scores, lower pain scores, and improved gait analysis with PEMF treatment when compared with controls.[37,38] In neurologic injuries, use of PEMF leads to quicker improvement, a more complete recovery, and enhanced pain control for small animal patients.[39–42]

Table 4
Co-analgesics in veterinary palliative care

Drug	Mechanism of Action	Indications	Cautions/Side Effects	Frequency and Dosing	Notes	References
Amantadine	• Antagonist at NMDA receptor (dorsal horn) • Dopamine receptor agonist	• Patients with maladaptive pain • Patients with osteoarthritis • Beneficial in human patients with traumatic brain injury • Neuroprotective lab animal studies with spinal cord injury	• Sensitive gastrointestinal tract/Bad taste, typically vomiting • Can be stimulatory, best dosed in the morning when Q24. • Cardiac arrhythmias	• Initially, 3-5 mg/kg Q24 • Can be increased to 3–5 mg/kg BID as indicated, more effective pharmacokinetics at this dose	• Often used in combination with anti-inflammatories or gabapentin-type drugs and can be used on a short term or long-term basis	• Loggini • Dogan • Lascelles • Norkus[13-16]
Pregabalin	• Inhibition of calcium channels in the dorsal horn of the spinal cord (similar to gabapentin) • Reduction in release of neurotransmitters, overall reduction of neuronal excitability	• Neuropathic Pain • IVDD • Syringomyelia • Chronic Pain • Inflammatory pain • Lack of response to gabapentin, or poor response	• Sedation • Ataxia • Potentially dose reduction in patients renal disease due to slower excretion (similar to gabapentin)	• 4 mg/kg PO BID dogs • 1–2 mg/kg BID cats	• More linear pharmacokinetics when compared to gabapentin as well as stronger binding and higher bioavailability make response more predictable • Available as generic which has reduced cost	• Esteban • Salazar • Schmierer • Thoefner • Quimby[17–20]

(continued on next page)

Table 4
(continued)

Drug	Mechanism of Action	Indications	Cautions/Side Effects	Frequency and Dosing	Notes	References
Tricyclic antidepressants (TCA)	• TCAs modulate reuptake of serotonin and noradrenaline enhancing inhibitory control in the central nervous system	• First line analgesic for the management of neuropathic pain in human patients	• Caution regarding effect on serotonin and other drugs that may also impact serotonin • Side effects: sedation, constipation, and urinary retention • Use in caution with patients who have arrhythmias or known seizure disorders	• Amitriptyline: 1–4 mg/kg once daily to TID after assessing patient response	• The impacts on anxiety may be independent from those that manage neuropathic pain as TCAs impact numerous other receptors	• Wood • Cashmore • Kondratenko[21–23]
Ketamine	• NMDA receptor antagonist • Modifying neuroplasticity in patients with depression, anxiety, and complex pain conditions	• Chronic and Maladaptive pain • Cancer pain • Neuropathic pain • Depression/Anxiety (humans)	• Caution/dose adjust in patients with known cardiac arrhythmias • Caution/dose adjust in patients with seizure disorders	• 0.25–5 mg/kg IV bolus followed by 2–10 mcg/kg/min gradually increased to highest tolerated dose for 4 h	• Infusion frequency depends on severity of pain and patient response • When used in a low dose infusions or injections is	• Orhurhu • Patil • Bergadano • Cohen[24–27]

		• Caution in patients with elevated intracranial pressure and elevated intraocular pressure	• 0.5 mg/kg SQ PRN (human dosing is daily to monthly)	• generally safe and well tolerated • Can be dosed via subcutaneous pump at home or as intermittent subcutaneous dosing	
Low Dose Naltrexone (LDN)	• Modulates neuronal-inflammation reducing the release of inflammatory mediators from glial cells • Temporary blockade of opiate receptors and upregulation of metenkephlin • Increased production of endorphins	• Adjunctive pain medication in patients with known inflammation in the nervous system, immune mediated disease, and those with maladaptive or neuropathic pain • Very few side effects at low doses and is generally well tolerated • Possible pruritus	• 0.1 mg/kg once daily in the evening, working up to TID in severely affected cases	• This small dose size does require compounding of this medication, according to compounding regulations within individual states	• Kim • White • Machado[28-30]
Polysulfated Glycosaminoglycan (PSGAG)	• Inhibition of catabolic enzymes within the joint • Reduction in prostaglandins • Increased synovial viscosity	• Osteoarthritis • Caution with patients with propensity for bleeding, can act as anticoagulant • Diarrhea, usually responsive to dose reduction	• 4.4 mg/kg intramuscular, twice weekly for 4 wk then can repeat this dosing as needed	• Authors prefer subcutaneous dosing	• Varcoe • Sevalla[31,32]

(continued on next page)

Table 4
(continued)

Drug	Mechanism of Action	Indications	Cautions/Side Effects	Frequency and Dosing	Notes	References
Lidocaine Patches	-Inhibition of sodium channels to stabilize nerve membranes • True nociception blockade	• Local Pain • Allodynia • Joint pain/osteoarthritis • Post operative/intervention (joint injection)	• Local skin irritation • Minima systemic absorption, so minimal risk of systemic toxicosis	• For chronic pain apply in rotating 12 h on 12 h off schedule	• Hair needs to be clipped for application	• Weil[33]

Table 5
Rehabilitation modalities for palliative care patients

Modality	Mechanism of Action	Indications	Cautions	Frequency and Dosing	Notes	Devices Available
PEMF Therapy	Generation of an electromagnetic field, when applied to tissues, alters calcium and calmodulin signaling to: • Reduce inflammation • Alter immune function • Decrease pain signaling • Upregulate fibro/osteoblasts	• Edema • Pain- Neurologic and Musculoskeletal • Wound healing • Nerve function • Bone healing and osteopenia	• Overall, tends to be very safe with relative cautions • Pregnancy due to unknown impacts • Open growth plates due to potential for calcification of bone • Active bleeding	• A minimum of 30–69 min daily • As recommended by manufacturer of specific products	• Wearable technology or dog beds can provide longer durations of treatment	• Beds and mats -Wearable rings/loops • Soft sided carriers for small animals • Wearable patches
Laser Therapy	Photobio-Modulation occurs when photons are absorbed by Cytochrome C in the electron transport chain and leads to: • Reduced inflammatory cascade • Reduced edema • Enhanced neurologic function	• Edema • Pain- Neurologic and Musculoskeletal • Wound Healing • Nerve function • Myofascial pain syndrome • Muscle tension	• Overall, tends to be very safe with relative cautions • Pregnancy due to unknown impacts • Open growth plates due to potential for heat or cell proliferation • Active bleeding • Certain types of neoplasia	• Daily to weekly treatments • Home therapy possible • Generally 2–4 J/cm^2 is an adequate dose • Excessive dosing can slow wound healing		• Class 3 and Class 4 lasers are typically used during in-clinic visits • Class 3 devices or LED devices can be safely used at home for interested clients

(continued on next page)

Table 5
(continued)

Modality	Mechanism of Action	Indications	Cautions	Frequency and Dosing	Notes	Devices Available
	• Enhanced circulation and angiogenesis • Upregulation of ATP • Wound healing via fibroblast migration					
Acupuncture	• Coupling of the acupuncture needles with underlying collagen leads to a physiologic pull that will in turn: -Cause neuromodulation of the CNS, PNS and ANS • Reduction in inflammatory mediators • Enhance fibroblasts and wound healing • Enhance organ function through somato-visceral feedback and modulation of the autonomic nervous system	• Pain- Neurologic and musculoskeletal and visceral • Change in appetite • Sarcopenia • Weakness • Nerve function • Myofascial pain syndrome • Muscle tension • Systemic disease- for example, renal, liver, cardiovascular, pulmonary and gastrointestinal disease or discomfort	• Overall, tends to be very safe with relative cautions • Coagulopathy or severely decreased platelets • Patient with severe anxiety or one that cannot settle down during a treatment	• Weekly, monthly or anywhere in between, depending on stage of palliative care, client's financial and temporal budget, client's educational needs and patient's response to acupuncture	• Regular acupuncture visits allow the veterinary professional time to connect with clients for education, to answer questions and help with quality of life assessments	• Must be performed in a clinical setting • "Dry needling" techniques can be done with care in geriatric patients • Acupuncture and electroacupuncture should always be done within the patient's comfort level • Carry a variety of needles from 0.16 mm to 0.20 mm needles for gentle but effective treatment

Shockwave Therapy	Tissue compression secondary to strong acoustic wave leads to: • Enhanced fibroblast and osteoblast activity • Upregulation of growth factors • Altered local nociceptor activity • Regional angiogenesis	• Pain- Neurologic and Musculoskeletal • Wound Healing • Myofascial pain syndrome • Muscle tension • Lumbosacral dysfunction • Tendinopathies • Degenerative joint disease	• Overall, tends to be safe with relative cautions that apply to high or very high energy units and settings • Directly over metal implants with high energy levels • Directly over lung fields with deep focal heads	• Every 2–4 wk as needed • Typically a longer lasting therapy, though when given in smaller/gentler doses as in palliative care, increased frequency may be preferable	• The type of machine and its parameters make it more applicable and gentler for palliative care, so that sedation and restraint aren't necessary	• Electrohydraulic • Electromagnetic • Piezoelectric • Radial
Therapeutic Exercise	Moderate-intensity exercise can: • Reduce pain • Enhance muscular proprioception by adding muscle spindles and Golgi Tendon organs • Reduce progression of sarcopenia • Improve mobility and independence by enhancing overall balance	• Weakness • Loss of mobility • Inability to rise • Difficulty with elimination • Pain- Neurologic and Musculoskeletal • Loss of conscious proprioception • Myofascial pain syndrome • Overly tight muscles	• Very safe, especially if done with support and proper education for clients • Swim with caution in patients who are too weak to hold their head well or have a serious limb injury • High impact and long duration exercise can increase soreness	• Two gentle sessions each week are likely enough to make a positive impact • Additional home sessions can be helpful	• Consider balance and strength work as core targets of therapeutic exercise • Endurance, build through fun activities like walks and play are also an excellent addition • Some gentle stretching and massage can also be a valuable part of a home exercise program	• Balance equipment will enhance outcomes for patients and make the practitioner's creativity more expansive, giving more, enjoyable exercises for a patient • Natural obstacles also work great, including a curb, a hill, a series of trees or shrubs, uneven rocks or a sandy spot to walk or dig

Table 6
Intra-articular injections for palliation of joint pain

Component	Goal	Duration of Effect	Cost	Notes
Hyaluronic Acid (HA)	• Increase intra-articular joint fluid viscosity • Analgesia	• Variable • 1 mo in severely affected joints • Up to 4–6 mo in humans	$-$$	• Higher molecular weight HA is superior but more expensive • Combined with other products, can enhance effect and longevity of those products
Triamcinolone	• Greatly reduce synovial inflammation	• Variable • Weeks to 1 month in severely affected patients • May be enough to allow other therapies to begin working	$	• Combined with other products, triamcinolone can reduce joint flare and post-injection pain • Generally discourage several repeat injections due to potential for cartilage damage
Polyacrylamide Gel	• Increase viscosity in joint fluid and improve cushion within joint	• Variable • Up to 24 mo in horses • No published data in canine patients	$$-$$$	• Published data is primarily in horses, though being used clinically by some in canine patients
Platelet Rich Plasma	• Reduce joint inflammation • Enhance health of surface cartilage within joint • Analgesia	• Variable • Weeks to 1 month in severely affected patients • Maybe better when combined with other therapies	$$-$$$	• May be positive impacted by combining with HA for a longer duration of effect • Leukocyte-poor or pure PRP are superior for joint health and preferable in preventing joint inflammation in delicate palliative care patients

				• Highly variable clinical product due to number of PRP systems on the market-look for third party validation
Stem Cell Therapy	• Slightly stronger reduction in joint inflammation when compared to PRP • Enhanced health of surface cartilage within joint • Analgesia • Regenerative effect on cartilage	• Variable • One month up to many months	$$$-$$$$	• Best when combined with other therapies to maximize longevity • Stem cells can be derived from bone marrow or adipose tissue • Strong immune-modulating component
Tin (117mSn) Stannic Colloid-Conversion-Electron Therapeutic Device	• Gamma radiation induces apoptosis of inflammatory cells and thereby reduced overall joint inflammation • Analgesia	• Variable • Up to 12 mo	$$$$-$$$$	• Primarily licensed for elbow OA • Radioactive nature means heavy sedation for injections and discussion with owners regarding safe patient handling post-injection • Extensive training and facility preparation before implementation

It is important to understand the safety and cautions of each modality when working with a delicate patient population affected by multiple disease processes. PEMF has demonstrated safety and potential therapeutic benefits for cancer patients. Not only does PEMF address their oncologic pain and inflammation, but the potential for slight anti-tumor benefits also exists.[43,44] Cardiovascular safety has also been demonstrated, with potential benefits including improvement in congestive heart failure and cardiac arrhythmias via PEMF's ability to modulate nitric oxide production and neuromodulation autonomic nervous system.[45,46]

Ultimately, PEMF is a great therapeutic tool for palliative care patients because of its low cost and good safety profile, while offering pain management, anti-inflammatory benefits, and healing to patients who utilize one of the convenient commercial applications.

Therapeutic Laser and Light Therapy

Therapeutic laser is generally used in clinical practice for analgesia, tissue healing, and enhancing neurologic function. Laser therapy is also frequently employed in the treatment of swelling, edema, and local inflammation, as it can attenuate inflammatory cytokine production and alter the influx of inflammatory cells into an injured region.[47–49] In addition to laser therapy, photobiomodulation with light-emitting diodes (LED) is gaining both popularity and understanding among the medical community.[49,50] Photobiomodulation, as all facets of laser and LED therapy are now called, can limit pharmaceutical use while improving comfort and healing for palliative care patients. Palliative care patients often have a combination of indications that would benefit from photobiomodulation, and as a result, their therapy can be time intensive. With palliative care patients, it may be worthwhile to consider at-home devices, which are convenient for pet owners and allow them to be involved in their pet's care. An appealing proposition for both the veterinary team and clients caring for a palliative care patient.

When discussing the indications for photobiomodulation in these patients, the treatment of self-inflicted wounds and pressure sores, musculoskeletal pain, neurologic degeneration, and inflammation come to mind. Laser's power to alter the inflammatory cascade, while upregulating fibroblast populations allow it to enhance collagen production and organization for both bone and soft tissue healing.[51] Photobiomodulation reduces both inflammatory pain, as well as neuropathic pain, making it an excellent tool for use in acute exacerbations of painful conditions, as well as for more chronic situations.[52]

In terms of safety, it is worth noting that excessive laser dosing has been shown to delay wound healing and reduce fibroblast metabolism in certain injury types, indicating that sometimes a lower-level approach may be superior.[53] Additionally, Alves and colleagues showed a superior reduction in inflammation in rats with joint injuries with the use of 50 mW therapy compared with 100 mW therapy.[47] Another commonly discussed safety topic for light therapy is its use in the presence of known or suspected neoplasia, as the ability of photobiomodulation to enhance cell proliferation could theoretically contribute to aggression in certain cancer types. In a recently published review, however, over 27 published human articles indicated little safety concern for cancer patients and worthwhile benefit for the treatment of cancer-treatment-related maladies.[54] As the data remain unclear, clinicians may want to exercise caution with laser treatment in neoplastic patients, but when addressing end-of-life concerns, photobiomodulation may provide more benefit than potential harm for a selection of patients.

Acupuncture

Acupuncture is a powerful modality that should not be overlooked in the palliative care setting. Its safety has been well established, while its efficacy for a myriad of painful and disease-related conditions is extensive in both human and veterinary literature. [55–60] Acupuncture is an essential tool for the treatment of chronic pain, neurologic degeneration, and systemic disease because, in addition to modulating pain, acupuncture can neuromodulate the autonomic nervous system, influencing visceral function through somato-visceral neural feedback loops.[61] An improved appetite, ease in labored breathing, improved glomerular filtration, and enhanced wound healing are just a few of the additional benefits a palliative care patient might reap from this modality.[62]

With a medical understanding of acupuncture, a clinician treats acupuncture points rich in nerves, nerve endings, blood vessels, fascia, and lymphatics, making them ideal therapeutic targets.[63] The interaction of the needle with the underlying structures is mediated by a tight coupling of the needle to the surrounding connective tissues, in which the practitioner's manipulation of the needle creates direct mechanical signaling and a cascade of cellular events that create local, regional, and systemic effects.[64] Fibroblast activation, mast cell degranulation, and the local activation of A1-adenosine receptors lead to many of the local and regional effects of acupuncture, which go on to stimulate TrpV receptors (selective calcium receptors involved in pain signaling), cannabinoid receptors, and more.[65] From these local effects ensue a series of changes in the dorsal horn of the spinal cord and the perceptual experience within the brain.[66]

Ultimately there is reduced pain perception, along with an endogenous downregulation of pain signaling in the spinal cord tracts, leading to more enhanced comfort for the treated patient. Acupuncture for geriatric and diseased patients should be a gentle and relaxing experience, enjoyed by both patient and client—a perfect addition to almost every palliative care treatment plan. It also offers a compelling aid to reduced doses of medications for complex, painful patients.

Extracorporeal Shockwave Therapy

Extracorporeal shockwave therapy, which was once best known for its role in lithotripsy, has found application in the realm of veterinary musculoskeletal pain and disease. The brief but intense pressurized acoustic waves emitted from a unit travel into tissues, and the resulting cascade of physiologic changes leads to significant therapeutic benefits. The mechanical compression that occurs causes angiogenesis, fibroblast/osteoblast activation, and the release of growth factors, which prove to be both healing and analgesic.[67]

There is both an immediate analgesic benefit, followed by a biphasic secondary analgesic effect weeks to months after a therapy session. Because this immediate analgesic benefit exists, shockwave is a modality well-suited to palliative care patients, who get the benefit of immediate analgesia as well as improved joint health for those with a longer life expectancy. Typical therapeutic targets include chronic degenerative stifle arthritis, painful shoulders and hips, arthritic or dysplastic elbows, and chronic lumbosacral disease.[68–70] With safety well established, and both short and long-term benefits for these patients in both comfort levels and tissue healing, shockwave therapy should be considered for every palliative care patient with degenerative musculoskeletal conditions or myofascial pain.

Therapeutic Exercise

Therapeutic exercise is at the core of a usual rehabilitation program, but in the case of palliative care, many times both practitioners and clients are hesitant to include therapeutic exercise in a patient's program. Although the benefits of continued movement are evident from abundant published data,[71] as patients get older and less mobile, sometimes clients feel that encouraging movement may be damaging or painful. On the contrary, moderate-intensity movement reduces pain and helps maintain mobility in humans,[72,73] which likely translates to small animal patients. Therapeutic exercise can be used for nearly every type of musculoskeletal and neurologic injury, and can also be helpful during recovery from illnesses such as pneumonia or gastrointestinal upset.

Therapeutic exercise for palliative care combines the adaptation of geriatric human approaches and individual patient modification to achieve enjoyable and productive exercises for each patient. By introducing voluntary, active weight-bearing and movement, therapeutic exercise will help maximize the well-being and comfort of palliative care patients. Incentivizing voluntary participation in therapeutic exercise with rewards improves those outcomes and enhances the experience for client and pet.

Two generalized goals for therapeutic exercise can be considered—proprioceptive exercise and strengthening exercise. Loss of balance and proprioception contributes to an inability to rise and loss of independence, which can be threatening to the quality of life for small animal patients. Resistance training, or weight-lifting, used to achieve strength training in humans is more challenging in animal patients, yet enhancing muscular strength is important. It can require a creative approach as the voluntary and repetitive participation of the patient is needed. Combined proprioceptive and strength exercises can reduce the progression of sarcopenia and enhance independent ambulation in both human and small animal populations, even only twice weekly, making this an achievable goal for most palliative care families.[74] Working on unstable and uneven surfaces, as well as using balance equipment, can enhance proprioception and reduce functional disability while building balance, strength, and endurance. Geriatric patients can also engage in isometric exercises and eccentric or concentric strength exercises, using the patient's body as resistance. Both proprioceptive and strength training help mitigate sarcopenia in aging patients, helping to prevent the progression of muscle loss, and the rising risk of further comorbid conditions. Like some of the other modalities, the incorporation of therapeutic exercises into the home and clinical palliative care programs is an important way to maintain mobility and independence for a small animal patient.

SUMMARY

Palliative rehabilitation is an incredibly rewarding discipline in which patient-centered care can lead a rehabilitation practitioner to work with clients to develop function-targeted goals for patients with terminal or progressive disease processes. Despite the progression of disease in these patients, the reward that can be realized from appropriate pain management, ongoing work on joint health, and a focus on the primary disabilities can be enormous. The combination of pharmaceuticals with rehabilitation modalities puts veterinary professionals in a unique position to truly enhance the quality of life for small animal patients and the family who cares about them.

CLINICS CARE POINTS

- Use of the disablement model encourages the practitioner to define the functional limitations and address them as part of their treatment plan, rather than focus on the underlying etiologies.

- A focus on exhaustive diagnostic testing can be counterproductive in palliative care patients. Treatment should not be withheld due to lack of diagnostics.
- Appropriate pain management requires assessment of the risk-benefit ratio for patients in palliative care, whose goals and outcomes require a proactive approach to prescribing medications to achieve a satisfying outcome for patients, clients, and clinicians.
- PEMF and photobiomodulation are useful for pain management and healing, with few contraindications, and are safe and readily available for home use.
- Acupuncture is an essential component of a treatment plan for geriatric patients with complex conditions because of its ability to impact the autonomic, somatic, and visceral nervous system.
- Shockwave is incredibly beneficial for arthritis and myofascial pain that accompanies aging in palliative care patients.
- Activity and therapeutic exercise should be a continued aspect of a patient's lifestyle, even as disability advances with age and the progression of the disease.

DISCLOSURE

The authors of this paper have no conflicts of interest and no disclosures to make.

REFERENCES

1. Bishop G, Cooney K, Cox S, et al. AAHA/IAAHPC End-of-Life Care Guidelines. J Am Anim Hosp Assoc 2016;52:341–56.
2. Cheville AL, Morrow M, Smith SR, et al. Integrating Function-Directed Treatments into Palliative Care. PM R 2017;9(9S2):335–46.
3. Verbrugge LM, Jette AM. The disablement process. Soc Sci Med 1994; 38(1):1–14.
4. Snyder AR, Parsons JT, Valovich McLeod TC, et al. Using disablement models and clinical outcomes assessment to enable evidence-based athletic training practice, part I: disablement models. J Athl Train 2008;43(4):428–36.
5. Poitras ME, Maltais ME, Bestard-Denommé L, et al. What are the effective elements in patient-centered and multimorbidity care? A scoping review. BMC Health Serv Res 2018;18(1):446.
6. Frye C, Carr BJ, Lenfest M, et al. Canine Geriatric Rehabilitation: Considerations and Strategies for Assessment, Functional Scoring, and Follow Up. Front Vet Sci 2022;9:842458.
7. Spitznagel MB, Carlson M. Caregiver Burden and Veterinary Client Well-Being. Vet Clin Small Anim 2019;49:431–44.
8. Liu Z, Heffernan C, Tan J. Caregiver burden: A concept analysis. Int J Nurs Sci 2020;7(4):438–45.
9. Gallagher-Thompson D, Robinson Shurgot G, Rider K, et al. Ethnicity, Stress, and Cortisol Function in Hispanic and Non-Hispanic White Women: A Preliminary Study of Family Dementia Caregivers and Noncaregivers. Am Jof Geriatr Psychiatry 2006;14(4):334–42.
10. Schulz R, Martire L. Family Caregiving of Persons With Dementia: Prevalence, Health Effects, and Support Strategies. The Am J Geriatr Psychiatry 2004; 12(3):240–9.
11. Peterson NW, Boyd JW, Moses L. Medical futility is commonly encountered in small animal clinical practice. J Am Vet Med Assoc 2022;260(12):1475–81.
12. Moore SA. Managing Neuropathic Pain in Dogs. Front Vet Sci 2016;3:12.

13. Loggini A, Tangonan R, El Ammar F, et al. The role of amantadine in cognitive recovery early after traumatic brain injury: A systematic review. Clin Neurol Neurosurg 2020;194:105815.

14. Dogan G, Karaca O. N-methyl-D-aspartate Receptor Antagonists may Ameliorate Spinal Cord Injury by Inhibiting Oxidative Stress: An Experimental Study in Rats. Turk Neurosurg 2020;30(1):60–8.

15. Lascelles BD, Gaynor JS, Smith ES, et al. Amantadine in a multimodal analgesic regimen for alleviation of refractory osteoarthritis pain in dogs. J Vet Intern Med 2008;22(1):53–9.

16. Norkus C, Rankin D, Warner M, et al. Pharmacokinetics of oral amantadine in greyhound dogs. J Vet Pharmacol Ther 2015;38(3):305–8.

17. Esteban MA, Dewey CW, Schwark WS, et al. Pharmacokinetics of Single-Dose Oral Pregabalin Administration in Normal Cats. Front Vet Sci 2018;5:136.

18. Salazar V, Dewey CW, Schwark W, et al. Pharmacokinetics of single-dose oral pregabalin administration in normal dogs. Vet Anaesth Analg 2009;36(6):574–80.

19. Thoefner MS, Skovgaard LT, McEvoy FJ, et al. Pregabalin alleviates clinical signs of syringomyelia-related central neuropathic pain in Cavalier King Charles Spaniel dogs: a randomized controlled trial. Vet Anaesth Analg 2020;47(2):238–48.

20. Quimby JM, Lorbach SK, Saffire A, et al. Serum concentrations of gabapentin in cats with chronic kidney disease [published online ahead of print, 2022 Feb 23]. J Feline Med Surg 2022. https://doi.org/10.1177/1098612X221077017. 1098612X221077017.

21. Wood H, Dickman A, Star A, et al. Updates in palliative care - overview and recent advancements in the pharmacological management of cancer pain. Clin Med (Lond) 2018;18(1):17–22.

22. Cashmore RG, Harcourt-Brown TR, Freeman PM, et al. Clinical diagnosis and treatment of suspected neuropathic pain in three dogs. Aust Vet J 2009;87(1): 45–50.

23. Kondratenko SN, Savelyeva MI, Kukes VG, et al. Experimental and Clinical Pharmacokinetics of Fluoxetine and Amitriptyline: Comparative Analysis and Possible Methods of Extrapolation. Bull Exp Biol Med 2019;167(3):356–62.

24. Orhurhu V, Orhurhu MS, Bhatia A, et al. Ketamine Infusions for Chronic Pain: A Systematic Review and Meta-analysis of Randomized Controlled Trials. Anesth Analg 2019;129(1):241–54.

25. Patil S, Anitescu M. Efficacy of outpatient ketamine infusions in refractory chronic pain syndromes: a 5-year retrospective analysis. Pain Med 2012;13(2):263–9.

26. Bergadano A, Andersen OK, Arendt-Nielsen L, et al. Plasma levels of a low-dose constant-rate-infusion of ketamine and its effect on single and repeated nociceptive stimuli in conscious dogs. Vet J 2009;182(2):252-260.

27. Cohen SP, Bhatia A, Buvanendran A, et al. Consensus Guidelines on the Use of Intravenous Ketamine Infusions for Chronic Pain From the American Society of Regional Anesthesia and Pain Medicine, the American Academy of Pain Medicine, and the American Society of Anesthesiologists. Reg Anesth Pain Med 2018;43(5):521–46.

28. Kim PS, Fishman MA. Low-Dose Naltrexone for Chronic Pain: Update and Systemic Review. Curr Pain Headache Rep 2020;24(10):64.

29. White SD. Naltrexone for treatment of acral lick dermatitis in dogs. J Am Vet Med Assoc 1990;196(7):1073–6.

30. Machado MC, da Costa-Neto JM, Portela RD, et al. The effect of naltrexone as a carboplatin chemotherapy-associated drug on the immune response, quality of

life and survival of dogs with mammary carcinoma. PLoS One 2018;13(10): e0204830.

31. Varcoe G, Tomlinson J, Manfredi J. Owner Perceptions of Long-Term Systemic Use of Subcutaneous Administration of Polysulfated Glycosaminoglycan. J Am Anim Hosp Assoc 2021;57(5):205–11.

32. Sevalla K, Todhunter RJ, Vernier-Singer M, et al. Effect of polysulfated glycosaminoglycan on DNA content and proteoglycan metabolism in normal and osteoarthritic canine articular cartilage explants. Vet Surg 2000;29(5):407–14.

33. Weil AB, Ko J, Inoue T. The use of lidocaine patches. Compend Contin Educ Vet 2007;29(4):208–16, published correction appears in Compend. table of contents. Dosage error in article text.

34. Wade B. A review of pulsed electromagnetic field (PEMF) mechanisms at a cellular level: a rationale for clinical use. Am J Health Res 2013;1(3):51–5.

35. Scardino MS, Swaim SF, Sartin EA, et al. Evaluation of treatment with a pulsed electromagnetic field on wound healing, clinicopathologic variables, and central nervous system activity of dogs. Am J Vet Res 1998;59(9):1177–81.

36. Ciombor DM, Aaron RK, Wang S, et al. Modification of osteoarthritis by pulsed electromagnetic field—a morphological study. Osteoarthritis and Cartilage 2003;11(6):455–62.

37. Pinna S, Landucci F, Tribuiani AM, et al. The effects of pulsed electromagnetic field in the treatment of osteoarthritis in dogs: clinical study. Pak Vet J 2013; 33(1):96–100.

38. Sullivan MO, Gordon-Evans WJ, Knap KE, et al. Randomized, controlled clinical trial evaluating the efficacy of pulsed signal therapy in dogs with osteoarthritis. Vet Surg 2013;42(3):250–4.

39. Alvarez LX, McCue J, Lam NK, et al. Effect of targeted pulsed electromagnetic field therapy on canine postoperative hemilaminectomy: a double-blind, randomized, placebo-controlled clinical trial. J Am Anim Hosp Assoc 2019;55(2):83–91.

40. Zidan N, Fenn J, Griffith E, et al. The effect of electromagnetic fields on postoperative pain and locomotor recovery in dogs with acute, severe thoracolumbar intervertebral disc extrusion: a randomized placebo-controlled, prospective clinical trial. J Neurotrauma 2018 Aug 1;35(15):1726–36.

41. Crowe MJ, Sun ZP, Battocletti JH, et al. Exposure to pulsed magnetic fields enhances motor recovery in cats after spinal cord injury. Spine 2003;28(24):2660–6.

42. Das S, Kumar S, Jain S, et al. Exposure to ELF-magnetic field promotes restoration of sensori-motor functions in adult rats with hemisection of thoracic spinal cord. Electromagn Biol Med 2012;31(3):180–94.

43. Muramatsu Y, Matsui T, Deie M, et al. Pulsed electromagnetic field stimulation promotes anti-cell proliferative activity in doxorubicin-treated mouse osteosarcoma cells. vivo 2017;31(1):61–8.

44. Xu W, Xie X, Wu H, et al. Pulsed electromagnetic therapy in cancer treatment: Progress and outlook. View 2022;20220029. https://onlinelibrary.wiley.com/doi/pdf/10.1002/VIW.20220029.

45. Sohinki D, Thomas J, Scherlag B, et al. Impact of low-level electromagnetic fields on the inducibility of atrial fibrillation in the electrophysiology laboratory. Heart Rhythm O2 2021;2(3):239–46.

46. Soltani D, Samimi S, Vasheghani-Farahani A, et al. Electromagnetic field therapy in cardiovascular diseases: A review of patents, clinically effective devices, and mechanism of therapeutic effects. Trends Cardiovasc Med 2021. https://doi.org/10.1016/j.tcm.2021.10.006. S1050-1738(21)00121-00123.

47. Alves AC, de Paula Vieira R, Leal-Junior EC, et al. Effect of low-level laser therapy on the expression of inflammatory mediators and on neutrophils and macrophages in acute joint inflammation. Arthritis Res Ther 2013;15(5):1.

48. Farivar S, Malekshahabi T, Shiari R. Biological effects of low level laser therapy. J Lasers Med Sci 2014;5(2):58.

49. Pigatto GR, Silva CS, Parizotto NA. Photobiomodulation therapy reduces acute pain and inflammation in mice. J Photochem Photobiol 2019;196(1):111513.

50. Heiskanen V, Hamblin MR. Photobiomodulation: lasers vs. light emitting diodes? Photochem Photobiol Sci 2018;17(8):1003–17.

51. Medrado AR, Pugliese LS, Reis SR, et al. Influence of low level laser therapy on wound healing and its biological action upon myofibroblasts. J Clin Laser Med Surg 2003;32(3):239–44.

52. de Andrade AL, Bossini PS, Parizotto NA. Use of low level laser therapy to control neuropathic pain: a systematic review. J Photochem Photobiol 2016;164(1):36–42.

53. Bjordal JM, Couppé C, Chow RT, et al. A systematic review of low level laser therapy with location-specific doses for pain from chronic joint disorders. Aust J Physiother 2003;49(2):107–16.

54. de Pauli Paglioni M, Araújo AL, Arboleda LP, et al. Tumor safety and side effects of photobiomodulation therapy used for prevention and management of cancer treatment toxicities. A systematic review. Oral Oncol 2019;93:21–8.

55. He Y, Guo X, May BH, et al. Clinical evidence for association of acupuncture and acupressure with improved cancer pain: a systematic review and meta-analysis. JAMA Oncol 2020;6(2):271–8.

56. Vickers AJ, Vertosick EA, Lewith G, et al, Acupuncture Trialists' Collaboration. Acupuncture for chronic pain: update of an individual patient data meta-analysis. J Pain 2018;19(5):455–74.

57. Witt CM, Brinkhaus B, Reinhold T, et al. Efficacy, effectiveness, safety and costs of acupuncture for chronic pain–results of a large research initiative. Acupuncture Med 2006;24(1):33–9.

58. Silva NE, Luna SP, Joaquim JG, et al. Effect of acupuncture on pain and quality of life in canine neurological and musculoskeletal diseases. Can Vet J 2017;58(9):941.

59. Chomsiriwat P, Ma A. Comparison of the Effects of Electro-acupuncture and Laser Acupuncture on Pain Relief and Joint Range of Motion in Dogs with Coxofemoral Degenerative Joint Disease. Am J Chin Med 2019;14(1):11–20.

60. Veit N. Acupuncture as palliative pain therapy for OCD in canine shoulder joint. Z für Ganzheitliche Tiermedizin 2013;27(2):46–8.

61. Yu Z. Neuromechanism of acupuncture regulating gastrointestinal motility. World J Gastroenterol 2020;26(23):3182–200.

62. Wen J, Chen X, Yang Y, et al. Acupuncture Medical Therapy and its Underlying Mechanisms: A Systematic Review. Am J Chin Med 2021;49(1):1–23.

63. Zhang ZJ, Wang XM, McAlonan GM. Neural acupuncture unit: a new concept for interpreting effects and mechanisms of acupuncture. Evid Based Complement Alternat Med 2012;2012:429412.

64. Langevin HM, Churchill DL, Cipolla MJ. Mechanical signaling through connective tissue: a mechanism for the therapeutic effect of acupuncture. FASEB J 2001;15(12):2275–82.

65. Trento MM, Moré AO, Duarte EC, et al. Peripheral receptors and neuromediators involved in the antihyperalgesic effects of acupuncture: a state-of-the-art review. Pflugers Arch 2021;473(4):573–93.

66. Fry LM, Neary SM, Sharrock J, et al. Acupuncture for analgesia in veterinary medicine. Top Companion Anim Med 2014;29(2):35–42.
67. Chamberlain GA, Colborne RG. A review of the cellular and molecular effects of extracorporeal shockwave therapy. Vet Comp Orthop Traumatol 2016;29(2): 99–107.
68. Dahlberg J, Fitch G, Evans RB, et al. The evaluation of extracorporeal shockwave therapy in naturally occurring osteoarthritis of the stifle joint in dogs. Vet Comp Orthop Traumatol 2005;18(3):147–52.
69. Becker W, Kowaleski MP, McCarthy RJ, et al. Extracorporeal shockwave therapy for shoulder lameness in dogs. J Am Anim Hosp Assoc 2015;51(1):15–9.
70. Mueller M, Bockstahler B, Skalicky M, et al. Effects of radial shockwave therapy on the limb function of dogs with hip osteoarthritis. Vet Rec 2007;160(22):762–5.
71. Millis DL, Ciuperca IA. Evidence for canine rehabilitation and physical therapy. Vet Clin North Am Small Anim Pract 2015;45(1):1–27.
72. Rocha TC, Ramos PD, Dias AG, et al. The effects of physical exercise on pain management in patients with knee osteoarthritis: A systematic review with metanalysis. Rev Bras Ortop 2020;2(55):509–17.
73. O'Connor SR, Tully MA, Ryan B, et al. Walking exercise for chronic musculoskeletal pain: systematic review and meta-analysis. Arch Phys Med Rehab 2015; 96(4):724–34.
74. Hassan BH, Hewitt J, Keogh JW, et al. Impact of resistance training on sarcopenia in nursing care facilities: A pilot study. Geriat Nurs 2016;37(2):116–21.

Moving?

Make sure your subscription moves with you!

To notify us of your new address, find your **Clinics Account Number** (located on your mailing label above your name), and contact customer service at:

Email: journalscustomerservice-usa@elsevier.com

800-654-2452 (subscribers in the U.S. & Canada)
314-447-8871 (subscribers outside of the U.S. & Canada)

Fax number: 314-447-8029

Elsevier Health Sciences Division
Subscription Customer Service
3251 Riverport Lane
Maryland Heights, MO 63043

*To ensure uninterrupted delivery of your subscription, please notify us at least 4 weeks in advance of move.

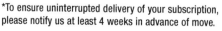

Printed and bound by CPI Group (UK) Ltd, Croydon, CR0 4YY

03/10/2024

01040473-0019